The Clean
in
14
DETOX

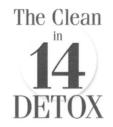

The Clean

in

14

DETOX

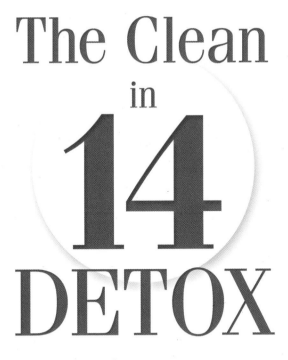

The 2-WEEK Plan to Melt Fat, Kick Cravings, and Increase Your Natural Energy

Melissa Costello

Health Communications, Inc.
Deerfield Beach, Florida

www.hcibooks.com

Disclaimer: The advice contained in this book is not intended as a substitute for the advice and/or medical care of the reader's physician. The reader should regularly consult with a physician in matters relating to his or her health. Any eating or exercise regimen should not be undertaken without consulting with the reader's physician.

Cataloging-in-Publication Data is available through the Library of Congress

ISBN-13: 978-0-7573-1784-2 (paperback)
ISBN-10: 0-7573-1784-7 (paperback)
ISBN-13: 978-0-7573-1785-9 (e-book)
ISBN-10: 0-7573-1785-5 (e-book)

HCI, its logos, and marks are trademarks of Health Communications, Inc.

Publisher: Health Communications, Inc.
        3201 S.W. 15th Street
        Deerfield Beach, FL 33442–8190

Photographer: Roy Dunn, www.roypix.com
Melissa Costello's hair styling: Denise Baker
Cover and interior design by Lawna Patterson Oldfield

Contents

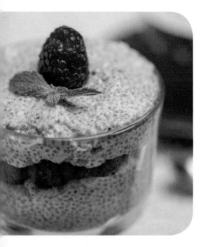

Breakfast and Shakes

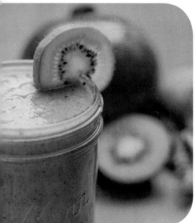

Other Shakes, Teas, and Comfort Treats

Snazzy and Satisfying Salads

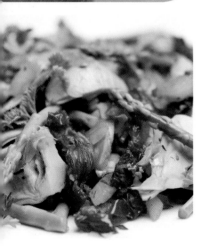

Slurp-Worthy Soups and Stews

Main Meals and Delightful Bowls

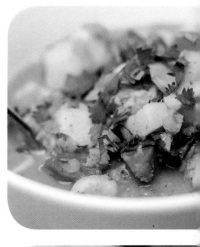

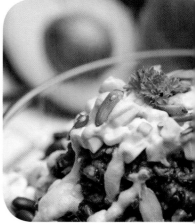

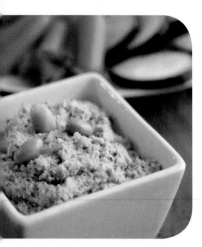

Delectable Dips for Snacking

Acknowledgments

Writing a book is not an easy task, and one that takes a lot of time, patience and nurturing. I want to thank those that offered me all of those things while I was creating this amazing, life-changing program.

To Allison Janse, Lawna Oldfield, and everyone at HCI who practiced extreme patience and understanding when I went way past my deadlines, and for working with me to create the most beautifully designed cleanse book on the market. To Jill and Amber, my very dear friends who provide unconditional love and support no matter what. To Alan for being a beautiful light of love in my life, if only for a short while, and for tirelessly chopping veggies and washing dishes on photo shoot day. To my dear friend, Roy, an amazing and very talented photographer, for bringing the Clean in 14 foods to life, and for putting up with my perfectionistic nit-picking. To my sweet friends, Sofia (9) and Ruby (5), for their exuberant spirits and their recipe contributions to the program. To Stacey, whose consistent soul-sisterhood and friendship provides sweet comfort in my life. To my brother Chuck, and sister-in-law, Ingvild for all their love and support. To my sweet Pumpkin Pie, my adorable pit-mix, who provides unconditional love, laughter and healing in my life (and an excuse for daily beach visits). To God and the Divine for always reminding me to trust, time and time again.

And a very special thanks to all my amazing clients for their commitment and dedication to their health and well-being. If it wasn't for you, I wouldn't be able to deliver my passion to the world.

Introduction

After writing my first book, *The Karma Chow Ultimate Cookbook*, and receiving loads of positive feedback—and people desiring more of my simple, delicious recipes—I knew it was time to up my game and bring my passion for food-based cleansing to the world.

Over the years, I have been blessed to be able to teach thousands of people how to cleanse their bodies and find optimal health through eating a plant-based, whole foods diet. I don't usually like to use the word "diet," but the truth is, by definition terms, this way of eating is a diet, but not the kind you are used to hearing about or participating in.

This way of eating is not about deprivation or starvation. Most diets consist of some form of calorie counting, weighing and measuring food, and major deprivation, where your body goes into starvation mode to drop weight—utterly painful, in my opinion. I know that severe calorie restriction can be helpful for a truly obese person to drop weight, but it's usually not done in a healthful manner, nor is it completely necessary to drop weight. Clean, plant-based eating will do all of that, along with a regular, lifelong exercise program. Weight loss is a definite byproduct of clean eating, and it can happen naturally without restriction.

One definition of diet in *Webster's* dictionary is, "The foods eaten, as by a particular person or group." Diet is also defined as "a particular selection of food, especially designed to improve a person's physical condition or to prevent or treat a disease."

Both of these definitions of diet are aligned with my philosophy of prevention and health through clean food. Eating delicious, nutrient-dense foods that provide your body with the

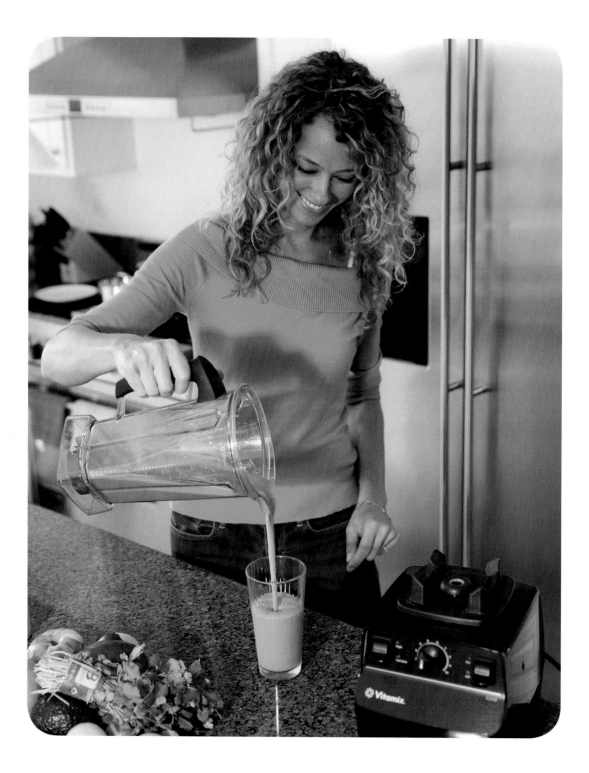

fuel it needs is the main focus of this program, along with some other exercises that will help you shift out of sabotaging behaviors and move into true freedom with food.

The reason I call it a "cleanse" is because you will be giving up certain foods and beverages that are of an addictive nature (i.e., coffee, refined sugar, alcohol, and processed foods—in other words, CRAP) that don't necessarily serve your body in reaching its optimal and balanced state, and you will not in the least feel like you are on a diet or that you are deprived. You will also be clearing sabotaging addictive patterns (SAP) out of your life so that you can continue on a healthy path once your cleanse is complete.

Eating delicious, nutrient-dense foods that provide your body with the fuel it needs is the main focus of this program, along with some other exercises that will help you shift out of sabotaging behaviors and move into true freedom with food.

You will break years of bad habits and find out what it's like to fuel your body versus eating just to eat. You will learn how to shift sabotaging behaviors that have kept you stuck in patterns of constantly having to go on a diet, and then falling off the wagon, and starting all over again. You will sleep better, lose weight, and find out what it's like to feel truly amazing and have energy!

Did you know that most people today walk around feeling crappy without even knowing it? They think it's the norm, because they don't know any better. Isn't that true of anything, really? We don't know until we know. That's why I felt compelled to bring the Clean in 14 Program to you, because I want you to experience what true health and vitality feels like. I want you to know that you can feel better. You can feel energetic, find your natural body weight, and discover a healthy eating balance in your life.

When I discuss healthy eating with my clients, the main aversion I most often come across is that they are afraid of failure or of not eating perfectly. Somehow, we've adopted a standard of perfection that we feel we need to live up to, and we think, *If I don't do it perfectly, what's the point?* So we just give up and throw all of our hard efforts out the window without keeping the bigger picture of optimal health and vitality in mind. Most of this mind-set comes from the media. We are bombarded every day with the next quick fix or new product that will help us feel better, look better, or "fix" what is broken—in other words, be/look perfect.

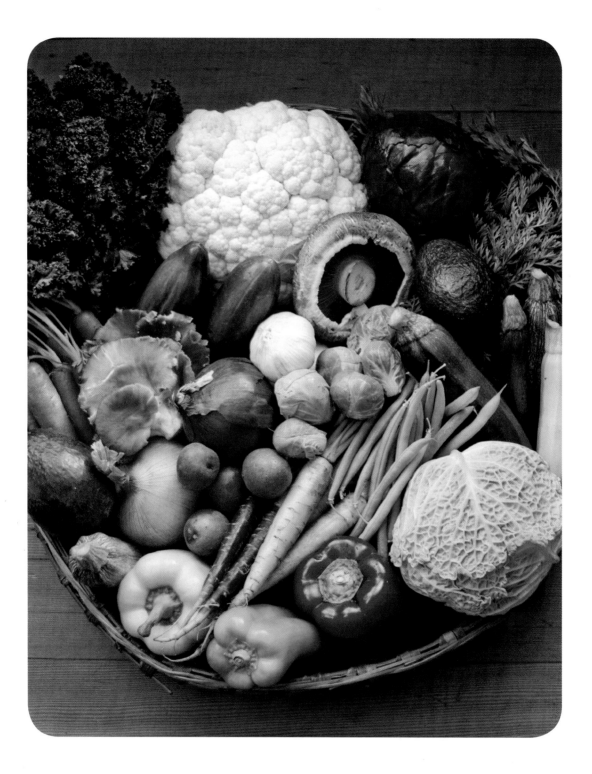

This program will provide a strong foundation for a lifetime of clean eating and feeling good. You will learn how to listen to and honor your body, how to eat consciously, how to manage the stress in life, and most important, how to take what you learn and confidently bring it forward into your daily life. The only true way to optimal health is by eating clean food, moving our bodies, getting enough rest, and managing our daily stressors and emotions.

The only true way to optimal health is by eating clean food, moving our bodies, getting enough rest, and managing our daily stressors and emotions.

We are all vastly different in many ways, and there is no one diet that is good for everyone. What this program will teach you is how to find the most optimal way of eating for you. It doesn't mean you need to be vegan, or even give up sugar for good; what it does mean is that you will be able to tune in to the needs of your body and feed it what will serve it best.

I know that embarking on a new journey can be scary, because it involves change. That is why I am providing you with everything you will need to be ready to start, including a week-long period of preparation, as well as how to bring forward what you learn during these next three weeks.

It's important that you read each section of this book carefully, as it's all critical to your journey. There is a lot of information provided here, and it may seem overwhelming at first, but I want you to understand exactly why your body needs to cleanse, as well as provide the platform to look deeper at some "bad" habits you may have picked up along the way that are not in your or your body's best interest. Think of it as an education. You are educating yourself so that you can make the best-informed decision for your health and your life.

I trust that the reason you picked up this book is because you are ready to make a change. And if what I've said so far scares you, then that means it's important to you, so continue on, my friend. Nothing worth *anything* was ever easy. It takes courage, commitment, and strength, and you have it all!

Are you ready? Here we go!

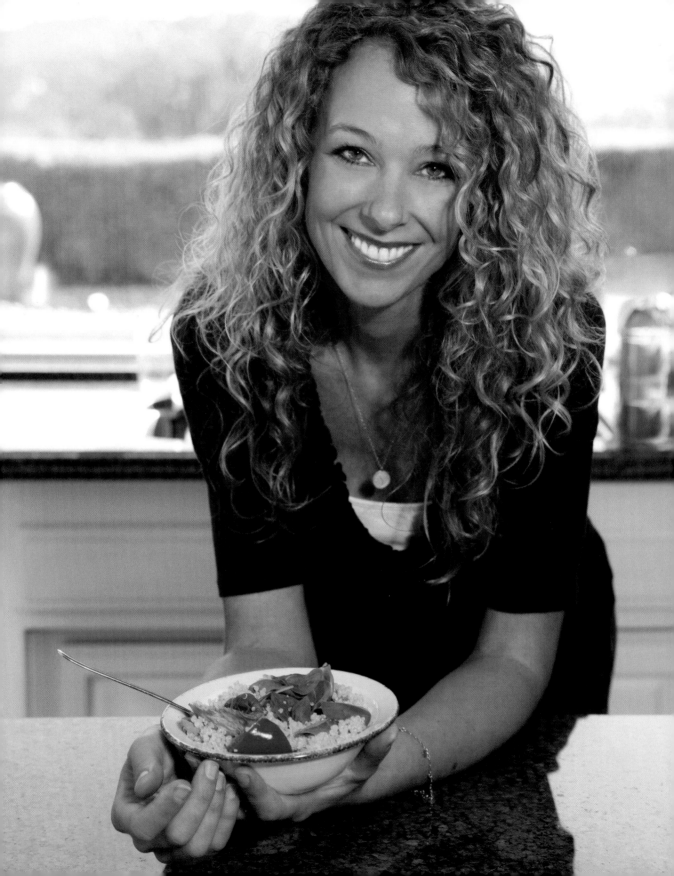

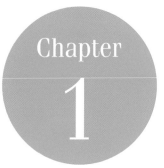

Getting Started: The Ins and Outs

You Can Do Anything for 14 Days!

Really, you can. Think about a time when you started a new venture, maybe a job, a workout routine, or learning to ride a horse. It took time. It took commitment. It took a plan, usually. And it took consistency. Maybe those things didn't feel as scary to you, but you went forward anyway. It was something you wanted, so you dove in. That's how this will be too.

I know you didn't pick up this book for the heck of it. Something inside must have been pulling you toward it, which in my eyes means you want to make a change. You want to learn how to feel better and to eat cleaner. You want optimal health and wellness. You want to stave off diseases. Think about 14 days in the big scheme of life and how small of a blip it is. Have you ever been on vacation for two weeks and it feels like it was three days? Well, that's how this program will feel too.

Yes, granted, you may experience some uncomfortable feelings at the beginning as your body detoxes and changes, but the result of amazing health and vitality in the long-term is what to keep in sight. Knowing that you're doing your body good for years to come and living a preventative lifestyle is beyond any quick fix or diet you can ever engage in.

But keep in mind: this is *not* a quick-fix diet or a magic pill. If that is what you are hoping for, then this program is not for you, and you might want to pass this book along to someone who is truly committed to changing their health for good. Or you can keep it in your back pocket for a future date when you feel ready to make a lifelong change. It's your call, but my guess is that you are ready *now*.

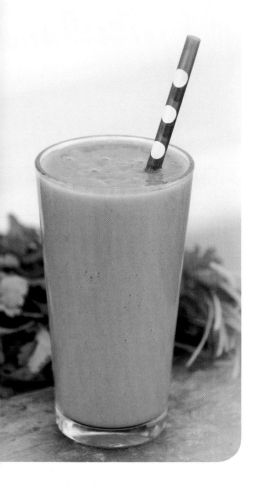

Do I Really Need to Cleanse?

Well, that depends. As I said in the introduction, we are all different. Our bodies vary vastly from person to person. The majority of people on the planet can benefit from some sort of seasonal cleansing every year, especially in the spring and fall.

Even if you consider yourself to be a healthy eater, chances are your body still needs a bit of support. Most people who think they are eating healthily get a serious eye-opening after doing this detox. This program will take you to the next level and show you where you can make even more positive changes to your diet for long-term benefits.

If you are an unhealthy eater and have never done a cleanse before, or don't know where to start, that's okay too. All of the information you need to be successful and change your eating habits is contained right here in this book. It's laid out in a simple plan so that you don't have to think too hard about it. All you have to do is take it step-by-step and day-by-day.

Over time our bodies can get gunked up with toxins from the food we eat, the air we breathe, and possibly even the water we drink. If you are someone who eats processed foods daily, drinks coffee, eats sugar, indulges in social or daily consumption of alcohol, drinks water out of plastic bottles or unfiltered water and eats out more than three times per week—which includes 99 percent of the U.S. population—then you are an awesome candidate for a cleanse.

This cleanse will provide your body with the nourishment it needs while cleaning out your organs and detoxifying your tissues, all by ingesting a lot of yummy, high-nutrient food.

I'm sure that you are probably familiar with some of the other cleanses out there that deprive you and starve you. Well, this cleanse will not do that. This cleanse will provide your body with the nourishment it needs while cleaning out your organs and detoxifying your tissues, all by ingesting a lot of yummy, high-nutrient food.

It will give you the foundation of a healthy, whole foods diet so that you know how to eat and what to put into your body to fuel it and give it energy without counting calories or measuring your food. How awesome is that?

Starvation Be Gone: The Power of Food-Based Cleansing

The reason I created a program using food to cleanse, versus relying on juices, supplements, or powders and potions, is because I want to teach you *how* to eat, and I want you to know what it really feels like to be satisfied by eating less food with higher nutrient content than you may be used to. Now when I say, "eat less," don't let that scare you. There are plenty of options available in this program, and you will never go hungry. The nutrient density and the delectable flavors of the food will keep you satisfied more than you may have ever felt before.

The foods offered in this program were specifically chosen because of their detoxifying and alkalizing qualities and nutrient density. This does not mean you have to follow the meal plan exactly, but you will receive the most benefit from it if you do. As you will learn, the more you read on and get into the heart of the program, there are a lot of foods you are allowed to eat on this cleanse, so feel free to be creative and add to my recipes if you'd like.

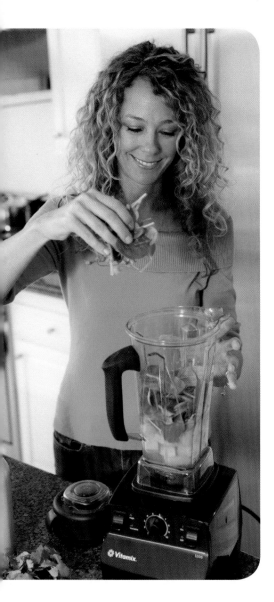

If you need to follow the plan to a T, that's okay too. However it works for you is best for you—let that be your mantra. You know yourself the best, so if you work best with an exact plan, take that route. If you want to be a little more loosey-goosey or creative with it all, yet stay within the parameters of the allowable foods, then go for it. Sometimes stepping out of the box can be extremely liberating, and if buying this book alone was a beginning of that for you, then bravo!

People are often confused about cleansing because there are so many different ones out there: juice feasting/fasting, the Master Cleanse or Lemonade Diet, water fasting, raw food detoxing, and more. The unfortunate thing about most of these cleanses (with the exception of the raw food detox) is that they are based on starvation and deprivation.

These cleanses starve your body of nutrients, which can be helpful in the detoxification process, but they are not necessarily good for your metabolism, adrenals, or hormones. Also, what usually seems to happen is that after people come off these detoxes, they go right back to their old habits and ways of eating. Sometimes they may even go off the deep end and eat "bad" foods that they weren't eating prior to cleansing. I remember doing a juice cleanse once, and all I craved was doughnuts. I don't even eat doughnuts—and hadn't for years—but my body was so deprived, I just wanted something fatty to fill me up.

Remember, the true key to vitality and wellness is finding what works for you. My guess is that you'd rather eat and feel satisfied versus not eat and feel deprived. Am I right? I will teach you how to use food as fuel and stop using it as a reward or something you turn to for comfort.

Cut the CRAP! Yes, You!

During the course of these 14 days (plus one prep week to get you cleanse-ready) you will be cutting the CRAP out of your life. This will give your body a chance to reset and recalibrate itself without any outside stimulants or toxins. Your metabolism will spark up and begin to rebalance itself too. Your blood sugar levels will even out, so you won't have as many cravings. You will tap into your natural source of energy. We all have it, but we often don't know it because it's been dumbed down by outside stimulants.

You might be wondering, what exactly is CRAP? While Chapter 5, "What to Avoid," gives a comprehensive list, here are the big four:

- Caffeine

- Refined sugars

- Alcohol

- Processed foods and fats

This CRAP (or what I also like to call "slow poisons") builds up in your system over a period of years and become toxic, causing your digestion to get out of balance and your energy to wane. They also create an acidic environment in the body, which can lead to many issues with your health, including skin problems, joint pain, inflammation, sugar cravings, lethargy, arthritis, clogged arteries, poor sleep, hormone imbalances, weight gain, and adult-onset diabetes, to name a few.

It's important to give your body a break from these foods/toxins so that it can find its own natural balance again. The cool part is that your body will start to transform from the inside out, and not only will you begin to feel better, but you will also start to drop weight. Our bodies are natural detoxifiers, but when they are clogged with CRAP, they can't detox without help. The foods in this program will do that. Once your body is regulated, it will be able to release toxins on its own, naturally, and weight will

> *Our bodies are natural detoxifiers, but when they are clogged with CRAP, they can't detox without help.*

begin to fall off. The inflammation in your body will cool off and you will begin to feel lighter and more energetic.

Although weight loss is a fantastic benefit of this cleanse, it's not the *only* benefit. You will go through many changes internally that you might not be able to see, and this will only be the beginning. Turning this way of eating into a long-term lifestyle will help your body come back to the natural vitality and health that it was born with.

Coffee: Why Do I Have to Give It Up?

Over the years, coffee has become a staple in the American diet. Wherever you go, there are coffee shops on every corner and in every town. Coffee has become a source of comfort, a source of energy, and a ritual of sorts. People drink it from morning to night, without even a thought of what it could be doing to their bodies—and sometimes it's just a vehicle for cream and sugar.

The truth about coffee is that if you consume it on a regular basis and feel like you can't get your day started without it, it most likely means you could have an addiction to it. If it scares you when you think about giving it up, that usually indicates some sort of attachment or false need for it. If someone told you that you had to give up kale, would you react the same? I think not. While coffee does have some good benefits, they don't outweigh the negative effects and what it can do to your endocrine system, especially if you drink multiple cups per day.

Coffee creates a false sense of energy. It wreaks havoc on the endocrine system. The caffeine creates a buzz in your body by raising your heart rate, releasing cortisol (our fight-or-flight belly fat–building response hormone), and releasing feel-good chemicals in your brain. I would think that any "substance" that did this would be something we'd want all the time. But that's where the addictive nature of coffee enters the picture.

I know it tastes good, and believe me, it's one of my favorite smells on the planet, but from my own personal journey, and knowing how hard coffee was to kick, it definitely felt like I was using a drug. I've had a love/hate affair with it all my life, and have gone back to it multiple times over the course of fifteen years, only to finally give it up totally because I felt like it was poisoning my system.

I recently did my own little experiment to see just how bad the effects of coffee were on me. I decided to go on a two-week coffee "bender" of sorts. One day I woke up and thought, *I want coffee, and I'm tired of depriving myself, so I am going to drink it and enjoy it.* This was the start of a very eye-opening experiment that led me to never wanting to even smell or drink the stuff again. I literally got so sick from it, my body rejected it, and I have learned to listen to my body when it gives me these types of signs.

Now mind you, over the last couple of years, I had been healing from adrenal fatigue and all sorts of hormone imbalances due to a tremendous amount of personal stress in my life that I wasn't managing well (yes, I am human too). It was imperative that I stay away from coffee at all costs to help my body heal, and I did this without issue.

But one particular day, I woke up wanting to go against everything I knew about coffee and how it could possibly harm me and give me a relapse. I thought to myself, *If I am enjoying it and believe it's good for me, what's the harm?* But that was just my ego and/or addiction speaking, and my body told me otherwise, thank goodness.

After two weeks of drinking freshly ground, organic, fair trade coffee every morning, my body shut down. I couldn't get out of bed. I felt like I had the worst hangover ever, and I don't even drink alcohol. This lasted for almost two weeks. I felt nauseous, had headaches, my digestion was off, and I had zero energy. This was a hugely eye-opening experience. All it took was two short weeks for my body to respond so sharply and resolutely.

Now, you might be saying to yourself, "Yes, well, I don't have adrenal fatigue and hormone imbalances," and while that may be true, the surest way to get adrenal fatigue is to continue to rely on coffee as your source of morning and afternoon energy. If you consume more than one cup of coffee per day, and you experience afternoon slumps, low energy, brain fog, digestive issues, headaches, poor sleep, and so on, coffee is most likely the culprit. It raises our blood sugar by dumping the stress hormone, cortisol, in our systems, and then we have a crash, which leaves us wanting more. It's acidic to our system, which creates a breeding ground for disease and digestive issues, and it disrupts our sleep patterns.

> If you consume more than one cup of coffee per day, and you experience afternoon slumps, low energy, brain fog, digestive issues, headaches, poor sleep, and so on, coffee is most likely the culprit.

Trust me, you can live without it. People who have done my 30-day Vital Life online cleanse program are blown away at how good they feel without it, how balanced their moods are, how much better they sleep, and how much more they get accomplished. It is a hard habit to break, but one that is worth breaking, once you feel all the positive results of life without it.

To save you from feeling totally deprived, I have given you a list of fun (and satisfying) alternatives that you can drink during this cleanse to replace the coffee in your life (see "Tea and Coffee Substitutes" in Chapter 7). These replacements are good for you, caffeine free, and offer comfort and ritual as well. It may feel different at first, but anytime there is a big change in our lives, we resist it until we continue forward and retrain ourselves to go a new direction. It takes time.

Refined Sugars: The Sweet and Poisonous Seduction

Sugar! It's gooey, sweet, seductive, and it has a hold on us! It's in almost every processed food sold, including mustard, ketchup, crackers, and peanut butter. It's the number one addiction in America today, and it's responsible for the massively growing obesity and type-2 diabetes epidemic! Did you know sugar is almost the exact molecular structure of cocaine and heroin?[1] Wow, that's a truly scary fact!

It has also been proven that eating sugar can depress the immune system for up to 6 hours afterward. Why do you think there is so much illness around holiday time? We ingest a bunch of sugar beginning at Halloween, and go right through to the New Year, thereby wreaking havoc on our immune system, leaving us vulnerable to the flu and other maladies. Every year, the flu epidemic seems to worsen, but part of the reason we may get so sick is because our immunity has been majorly compromised.

Food today is scientifically formulated to make us want more. As Dr. David Kessler explains in his book, *The End of Overeating: Taking Control of the Insatiable American Appetite*, scientists in the food industry are formulating food with the perfect combination of sugar and fat that releases feel-good chemicals in our brain, which changes our brain chemistry and makes it biologically addictive, so we want more and more.

---

1 Sugar Is Like Heroin. www.ncbi.nlm.nih.gov/pmc/articles/PMC2235907/

I recently went to an event where I was hired to cook for a group of people, and the host was a food scientist for a very popular fast-food chain. Really? You need a food scientist? Why? Why do you think?

Eating white, processed sugar or high-fructose corn syrup creates a perpetual cycle in our bodies that leads to more and more cravings. Why else would we not be able to pass by a dessert table without indulging? Sugar begets sugar, and so on. You get the idea. It has similar qualities as coffee, in the cycle of highs and lows, and it's even more addictive in nature. It's almost impossible to avoid, and remember, all sugars are not created equal. Sugar hides incognito in many foods with fancy names like "evaporated cane juice," "corn sugar," "cane syrup," and more.

Sugar! It's gooey, sweet, seductive, and it has a hold on us! It's in almost every processed food sold, including mustard, ketchup, crackers, and peanut butter. It's the number one addiction in America today, and it's responsible for the massively growing obesity and type-2 diabetes epidemic!

As you go through this cleanse, you will be allowed to have small amounts of low-glycemic, natural sweeteners and fruits with natural sugars. You will learn a lot about how your body feels without processed, high-glycemic sugars and what they can do to your mood. Did you know that refined sugars can even be a cause of depression? I do believe that we need sugar to survive. It feeds our muscles after a workout and can give us energy, if we ingest it in a healthy form. Our brain also needs a certain amount of sugar to function optimally too. But the problem is that we often overdo it and don't know how or when to stop. Most Americans ingest about 22 teaspoons of sugar a day, or 150 to 156 pounds of sugar per year. Yes, pounds! And most of it turns immediately to fat. To learn more about sugar addiction and the detrimental effects of sugar to your body, check out the classic book *Sugar Blues* by William Dufty.

Alcohol: Stress Reliever or Depressant?

People usually turn to alcohol as a way to reduce stress or wind down after a long, hard day. I think having a cocktail, beer, or glass of wine once or twice a week is okay, but most people tend to go overboard and drink every night and/or use alcohol to avoid problems or uncomfortable feelings.

From a physical standpoint, alcohol is also a depressant, just like sugar. It depletes serotonin levels over a period of time, which can lead to depression. Also, alcohol basically converts to pure sugar in your system, so it's responsible for weight gain, mood swings, and sugar highs and lows, which makes it hard to give up.

I am not saying you can never enjoy a drink again, but maybe it would be a good time to look at your drinking habits, if you have them, and question how you use alcohol, even if it's as a stress reliever. There are many other ways to relieve stress that are good for you rather than turning to a cocktail (see the "Impeccable Self-Care" list on p. 23). It's all about finding the balance that works for you. You may also find that when you give up drinking, you sleep more deeply and soundly. Your energy levels will increase too, especially in the morning.

Processed Foods and Fats (including Gluten Products)

As I explained in the introduction, processed foods are now created chemically by scientists to contain the perfect combination of sugar, salt, and fat. This combination tricks your brain and helps to release all those feel-good chemicals that leave you wanting more.

I know that if I dip my hands into a bag of a certain brand of potato chips that are oh so crispy, crunchy, and good, I can't stop at one or even 10. I almost have to finish the whole bag. It's like I am an addict and I can't control myself. I am not usually like this with food, except when it comes to processed foods, which is why I do my best to only indulge in them on rare occasions.

If you walk into a grocery store today, or any superstore with food, the majority of the food on the shelves was created in a lab, by a scientist, who was hired to put together the perfect combo of the trio mentioned above. There are brightly colored boxes with cartoon faces, bottles filled with neon-glowing dyed liquids, and sugar-laden treats all over the place. I am always appalled by the smell in a regular-type grocery store, and how it smells more like chemicals than real, fresh food.

America lives on processed foods. Why? Because it's convenient and easy. But convenient doesn't always mean healthy. And unfortunately, much of our society would rather choose convenience over health. Also, processed foods can be offered at a much cheaper price than true whole foods, because they are created in bulk in a lab by major corporations, and people buy it because they think they cannot afford to eat better. Sadly, this is a huge misconception. If you are eating for prevention, spending the money now is much better than spending it down the road when you are sick and obese. And you get much more bang for your buck when you are buying whole, high-nutrient foods. You

Processed foods are now created chemically by scientists to contain the perfect combination of sugar, salt, and fat. This combination tricks your brain and helps to release all those feel-good chemicals that leave you wanting more.

are feeding and fueling your body versus ingesting foods with not much nutritional value at all. You will also need to eat less, so you will save money doing that. And giving up daily habits, such as getting your favorite latte or a cocktail every night at happy hour, will save you tons of money as well. Think of it as an investment in yourself and your health. You are investing in your life *now*, versus waiting to be a victim of some illness or disease that takes over your life later on.

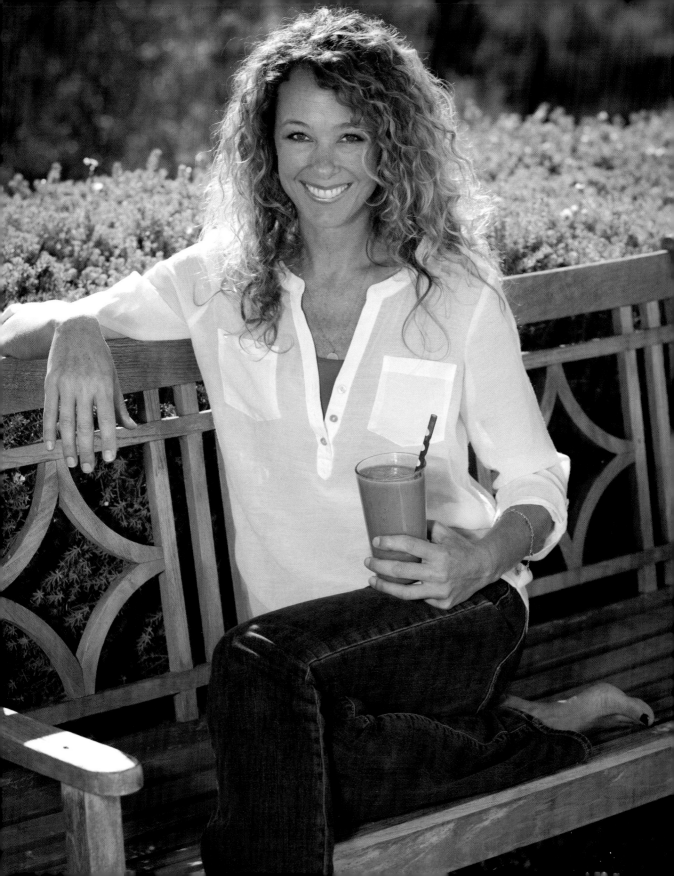

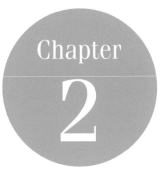

10 Basic Principles to Cleanse–and Live–By

During the 14-day program, you will be following 10 basic principles that will not only serve you during the cleanse but will also serve you for the rest of your life. You can use these principles daily, even after the cleanse is over. Turn them into your bible for healthy, balanced living. I've broken down each principle into detail so that you can dig in to each one and understand why they are so important for the 14-day cleansing process and beyond.

❶ Eat Good, Clean, Whole Foods

As I've related earlier in this book, eating clean, whole, unprocessed foods is going to support your body in the detox process, as well as nourish it with nutrients it may be missing out on. The more high-nutrient, whole foods we eat, the cleaner and more balanced our body becomes. This is essential to longevity, health, and sustained energy, as well as mood balance and deeper sleep. Eating clean will also reduce stress on your body, and help your digestive tract to work optimally. I have provided you with plenty of options of whole foods to eat during this program, so you won't have to worry about guessing.

❷ Hydrate, Hydrate, Hydrate

Drinking plenty of filtered, non-plastic bottled water is essential to the cleansing process. Staying hydrated will keep your body supple, as well as support it in detoxing naturally. Our body is mostly made up of water, so you want to be sure you are drinking at least a half-ounce per each pound of body weight. You can drink more if you desire, as it will support you in flushing

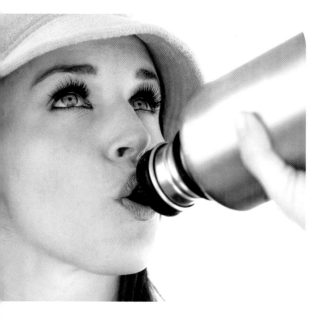

your internal organs and helping your digestive process be as smooth as possible. Water is one of the basic essentials that helps to keep us alive, along with sleep, food, and oxygen. It is a must that you stay well hydrated during this program which will keep you energized, and also help to prevent constipation as well.

Make sure to carry a water bottle with you everywhere you go. Portable bottles are best. I like stainless steel or BPA-free plastic ones. I usually keep one in my purse, one in my car, and one on my desk, so I know that I always have water wherever I go. Remember, being prepared is key!

❸ Move It and Use It

Moving your body during this program will be one of the key elements to your cleansing process. Exercise helps keep things moving, literally! The key here is to find the things you love to do that keep you active and to truly tune in to the needs of your body. If you don't know what your body needs yet, you will learn as you try new things and your body gets cleaner during the program. I am not saying you have to do hard-core workouts, but it's important that you move your body every day for at least 20–30 minutes.

If you are an avid exerciser, you may want to pare it back a bit in the first couple days. I know this may be hard, but part of this program is learning how to tune in to the needs of your body and what it is telling you. If you are tired, rest. If you are achy, take a bath or do some light stretching. Pounding your body when it needs to rest will just create more toxins and inflammation in your system and prevent your body from doing what it needs to do.

If you do not exercise regularly, it's important you move your body in some way every day for at least 15–20 minutes, even if it's a leisurely walk outside or on a treadmill. This will help your body release toxins and cleanse itself. Make sure to move your arms, put some music on, and go with it. You will get stronger and stronger each day and will be able to do more, but be sure to mix it up for best effect and to avoid boredom.

Yoga is a really good form of exercise to do during this cleanse, as well as cycling, dancing, interval training, rebounding, and brisk walking. If you are going to lift weights, do it at about 50 percent of what you normally would. It's best to take it easy during the detox phase of the program, when your body is working hard to release toxins. Everyone is different, so it could only be one day, or it could be three days. Whatever the length of the detox process for you, this is a time to be gentle on yourself and rest as much as you need to.

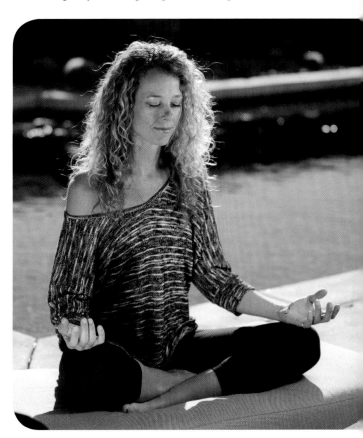

Remember, your body is working hard internally during these 14 days, so you want to be kind and gentle with it, not push it over the limit. It may be hard for you to cut back, but remember the benefits you will receive in the long term.

④ Sleep and Rest

Sleep and rest are extremely important during this program so that your body can recover and repair. When we sleep at night, our body goes into healing and mending mode. There is a lot going on internally, and I want you to get all the amazing benefits of this cleanse, so do your best to go to bed by 10:00 PM each night and stay away from any electronics at least one hour before bed (two hours is even better).

Getting seven to nine hours of uninterrupted sleep per night is the best source of stress management and healing for your body. This cleanse is void of the things that can disrupt sleep cycles, such as coffee and sugar. And it is chock-full of things that will support your sleep, such as good food, exercise, stress reduction, and self-care.

Resting is also a very important part of this program, which is different from the sleep you get at night. Taking naps if you have time will help you to heal and recover as well. Even if you can close your eyes for 15 minutes and let your mind drift, it will be very helpful in supporting you through the length of the program. Too often we push through when we don't have to, running on adrenaline, which taxes our body and wears it down. There is always a way to find 10–15 minutes in the day to get some quiet time to shut your eyes, so *do it!* You can even do the morning guided meditation in the middle of the day to reinvigorate yourself. Meditating can be more restorative and more restful than actual sleep.

⑤ Impeccable Self-Care

Taking impeccable care of yourself every day in an intentional way will help you feel good and give you the energy to show up and be more present for others in your life. I cannot stress this enough. This is why in the beginning of the book I suggested that you choose a time when your calendar can be cleared as best as possible. I understand that we are all busy and have things going on, but choosing a time when you can free up extra time will be extremely supportive to your process.

Your body will be going through a lot of change, and you want to allow it the space to do that by treating it with care. You will also want space to work with/through any emotions that surface during this process. By engaging in the evening ritual, you will help shift and release any patterns that are becoming more and more apparent to you. Here is a short list of my favorite Impeccable Self-Care activities. I also offer more in the daily exercises later in the book. Remember, taking care of yourself doesn't have to be a burden or an all-day affair. Take 10 to 15 minutes for yourself doing something that feels good to your soul and I promise you will feel a whole lot better as you go through this process.

IMPECCABLE SELF-CARE TO-DOS:

- Long hot Epsom salts bath
- Read your favorite book before bed
- Listen to your favorite music and dance around
- Lay in Savasana (Corpse Pose) for 5 minutes
- Visit the ocean and dig your toes in the sand
- Play a game
- Meditate for 5–10 minutes
- Play with your pet
- Watch a funny movie and laugh out loud
- Go to the mountains and hug a tree
- Journal or use Flow and Go writing
- Do something creative like draw, paint or take photos
- Call someone you love
- Visit a museum or other place of interest

⑥ Eat Consciously

Conscious eating means that we pay attention and *slow down* when we eat. It's all part of the Three W's (why you eat, when you eat, and what you eat), which we'll look at in more detail later. Oftentimes we eat on the go, in the car, or while we are running out the door. This doesn't give our body a chance to get the real benefit from all the nutrients we are ingesting. It disrupts our digestive system as well and makes it work overtime. It also disconnects us from our food, which can be detrimental to our health over time, meaning we are not paying attention to what is going in our body.

Conscious eating means sitting down to a meal, breathing, and taking space between bites. Make your mealtimes a ritual of fueling your body with nourishing food versus shoveling food down your throat as fast as possible just to get to dessert. The slower you eat, the more you can tune in to your body and feel when/if it is satisfied. You only want to eat until you feel *satisfied* and not *full*. This may take some time and practice to know when you are satisfied, because you may have been eating so unconsciously up until now, that your body doesn't even have a clue about how to calibrate itself. Be patient and look for subtle clues. My first clue is usually when I take a deep breath or sigh while eating. That is how I know I am almost to that point of satisfaction. I do my best to stop and give my food time to digest. I recognize that I

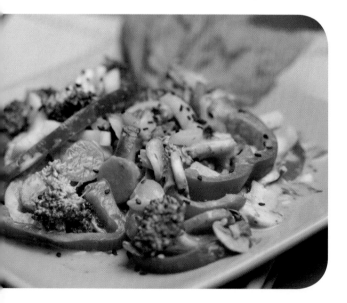

can always go back and eat more later if I am still hungry. Once you are full, it's too late. Your stomach is stretched to its max or beyond, and your food has nowhere to go. Your digestion cannot work how it's meant to. Now it's on overdrive and not fully absorbing the nutrients from your food. This can also cause acid reflux and a sluggish digestive system. Savor your food, taste it, enjoy it. Relish in the bounty of flavors and the fact that you have delicious, healthy food on your table, that you made and is filled with nutrients to fuel your body.

❼ Be Intentional

Being intentional means you are aware of your daily actions and that you are living on purpose, not from a place of complacency or passively letting life happen to you. You are making life happen, and you have an end goal in sight.

Committing to yourself during this journey might be the most powerful thing you can do. And if you write it down and say it out loud, it will be even more powerful. I know this sounds cliché, but when we live from an intentional place we have more of a chance of succeeding and following through with our commitments to ourselves. An even more effective plan is to share your commitment with another. Maybe there is someone you are close to who you can share your journey with who will help to lovingly hold you accountable.

I'm a big believer in tough love, because I feel that all too often we will let ourselves off the hook if something feels too hard or uncomfortable. A little tough love from someone who cares about you—or even a pep talk from yourself—can help you move through the SAP that has been holding you back. The SAP that has been ingrained in your brain and wormed its way into your everyday life so that you don't succeed in whatever you set out to accomplish for yourself needs to be defeated. And I provide you plenty of opportunity to do just that in the pages that follow.

❽ Ritual Building

Rituals help us stay balanced and on track. By starting and sticking to rituals, our life can open up to many other possibilities and positive life experiences. Human beings thrive on ritual and structure. Each day you will be given a morning and evening ritual that will help you get into a routine during the two-week

> **To Make Lemon Water**
> Heat 8 ounces of water in a kettle to almost boiling. Add the juice of a quarter of a fresh lemon.

cleanse. Set aside 20 minutes every morning before the kids get up (if you have them), and before your day gets started, to focus on the morning action items. These will include sipping a cup of hot lemon water, practicing deep breathing, reading your intention, reading an affirmation, and journaling. Each morning ritual will be pretty much the same, but you do not want to skip it, because it will set you up for success during the rest of the day.

Each evening, set aside 20 minutes before you go to bed to complete the activities listed, which will include journal activities and relaxing and unwinding. You can even do your ritual while sitting in bed, but make sure to allow for the full 20 minutes. Some activities won't take a full 20 minutes, but set this time aside anyway as a way to wind down and honor yourself. Practicing this ritual will help you reflect on the events of the day and sleep more soundly.

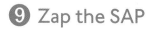 Zap the SAP

Becoming aware of and shifting long-term habits and patterns will provide a sense of freedom and openness. Each day of the program you will be given assignments in the morning and the evening that will be part of your ritual. These exercises will help you begin to look at, become aware of, and work through any SAP from the past—or that you are currently dealing with—that may be undermining your efforts to be healthy, lose weight, or eat well.

Not only will these tasks be very helpful in your process during the cleanse, but they will play an important role in setting up a foundation for you post-cleanse (see Chapter 10). You will examine your behaviors, where they stem from, and how they are (or are not) currently serving you. This might actually be the hardest part of the program, as I mentioned earlier, because it gets into the nitty-gritty of how you operate, and sometimes that can be scary and hard to look at. But just remember, you have the power within you to do anything, and with the support, education, and tools I am providing, there are no more excuses!

🔟 Let It Flow; Let It Go

"Flow and Go Writing" is a very useful tool that we'll be using throughout the cleanse. Writing down your thoughts in a steady stream of consciousness can help you clear the SAP, as well as release stress (see a more detailed definition of Flow and Go Writing in "Action Items for Day 1" in Chapter 8). Do not skip this process! It can provide huge insight for you—and emotional support as you go through the detox. Sometimes strong emotions can be released along with physical toxins throughout the detox process, which can take people by surprise. You may feel inundated with emotions of sadness, anger, or overwhelm. This is completely normal, and this is why it is crucial to use this tool, as it will help you clear anything that may be holding you back in life.

Since you need roughly 40 minutes total each day to participate in the exercises, write this time on your calendar and block it off (this time does not include your daily exercise/body movement). Some days, your task will be as simple as doing 10 minutes of deep breathing, while other days it will be more involved. Each task/exercise will be explained on each day of the program under daily rituals.

Writing down your thoughts in a steady stream of consciousness can help you clear the SAP, as well as release stress.

If you cannot find 40 minutes in your day to give to yourself, I highly recommend you reassess and reprioritize your life. When you don't make time to take care of yourself because you're burning the candle at both ends and eating poorly, you may take your stress out on others, which can create resentment. This is another way that disease can manifest in the body. It's all connected.

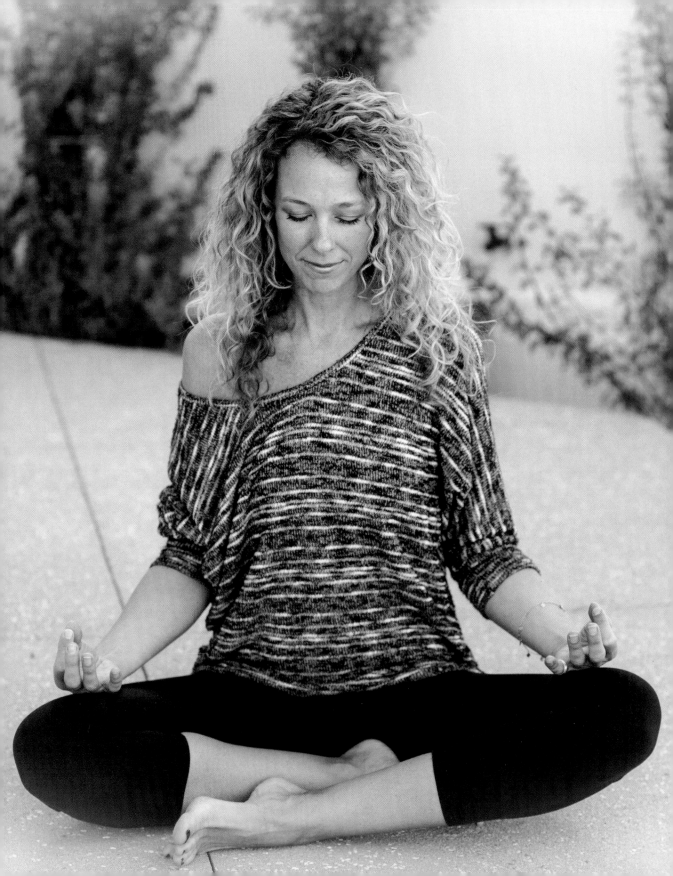

Your Questions Answered

What If I Don't Do It Perfectly? Will I Fail?

I mentioned earlier that sometimes when people hear the word *cleanse*, their body tenses up. What I have come to know is this: Most people are so worried about not doing it perfectly that they'd rather not do it at all. They feel that they might not be able to follow it perfectly, or in other words, they will *fail*. If this is your mind-set, I am here to tell you to *let that go . . . now!* Perfection doesn't exist, and even if you did follow the plan to an absolute T, there is no way you could do it perfectly, because your experience and outcome will be different than everyone else's, so you can see how there is no perfect way. It's individual and based on you, your body, and many other factors.

My mantra is, and has always been, "Progress, Not Perfection." I learned this from my years in 12-step programs, and it has helped me to focus on the progress I make each day in my life, not only with my diet but in all areas. Progress means we are changing for the better and getting a handle on something we may have not had a handle on before. It's all about taking one step at a time, which in my eyes *is* progress.

So although you will need to plan a bit while on this cleanse, I want you to take it one step and one minute at a time. Stay present and focused on yourself, your body, and the way you feel from moment to moment. This will teach you a lot. This will teach you not to get ahead of yourself and to really enjoy what's in front of you, whether that is chopping an onion or writing in your journal.

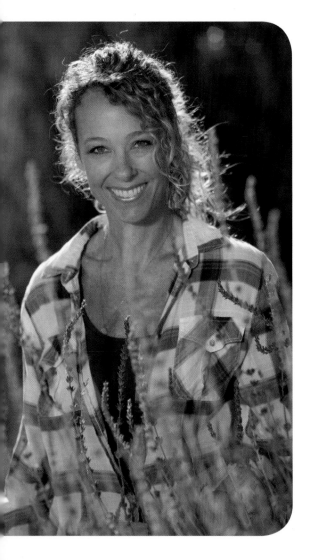

Will I Be a Social Outcast?

Another fear that many people have when starting a cleanse is that they will be social outcasts, or not be able to have any fun with their friends. This is where my tough love nature comes in and says to you, "Get honest with yourself. It's *only* 14 days out of your life, and if you can't commit to your health and well-being for 14 days, then you might as well throw this book out the window—and quite possibly your health too."

I know this may sound harsh, but the truth is, the fun is *not* going anywhere, and your friends, if they are your true friends, will understand and not give you a hard time. In fact, they will cheer you on and support you if they are your true friends. Some may even join you on the journey! You can forego booze and partying for two weeks, and even eating out. Health is made in your kitchen, not the kitchen of some restaurant or steak house. If you truly want to be healthy—and committed to having an awesome life—then you will do what it takes to achieve that.

Being social is important, and you can still be social, but maybe in a different way than what you or your friends have been used to. Who knows, you may even realize after the 14 days are complete that you don't want to do, eat, or drink the things you did before because you are feeling so darn good. Your friends may be upset and razz you a bit, but remember what I said: if they are your true friends, they will support you and understand, no matter what.

Being social is important, and you can still be social, but maybe in a different way than what you or your friends have been used to.

Whenever I am embarking on a new journey, or a big change in my life, I always ask the people closest to me for their support and help. It's really important to ask for what you need, and remember, people will only give you a hard time if they are afraid *they* have to change. It has nothing to do with you. It's a projection of their own fear of change and failure. You never need to defend yourself, and if your friends do not support you, then you have some important decisions to make about your life and the people you have kept company with up until now.

When I first began practicing yoga, my body felt so amazing, it just naturally craved healthier foods. I even stopped drinking alcohol all together, because it just didn't feel like it was in alignment anymore with my highest and healthiest self. This may happen to you, too. When you start to turn in a healthier direction, a lot of other things in your life could possibly start to fall away, including friends that may be toxic, too dramatic, or unhealthy.

Why Animal Free?

As you may have noticed, this program is completely vegan. I am not trying to turn you into a vegan, but what I do know is that our body needs a break from ingesting animal products. Animal products are very heavy in the system and take a long time to break down. They cause undue stress on the digestive tract and can clog it up.

Eating meat, eggs, and fish can cause mucus to build up in the intestinal tract, which makes it sluggish. When our digestion is off, our whole body is off. Our health starts in our digestive tract, so the key of this cleanse is to get your digestion back on track so that your metabolism and health can follow suit.

Animal products also tend to be high in saturated fat and cholesterol, so they contribute to many other diseases as well. To learn more about the effects of eating animal products, and what the demand for animal products does to the environment, I highly recommend watching any of the great documentaries out there, such as *Food Inc.*, *Forks over Knives*, or *Fat, Sick, and Nearly Dead.* I also recommend reading *Eating Animals* by Jonathan Safran Foer for a deeper look at the farming industry and where your meat, chicken, and fish are really coming from. If this doesn't interest you, that's okay. Just know that giving your body a break for these 14 days will benefit your journey to optimum health immensely.

Where Will I Get My Protein?

This is the first question I get asked when I tell people I am a vegan. It actually makes me chuckle a little, because the truth is, most Americans are overeating protein daily and getting *too much* animal protein in their diet. This can cause a buildup of ketones in the body, which can lead to ketosis, which is protein toxicity. Having too much protein is really hard on your kidneys and other organs.

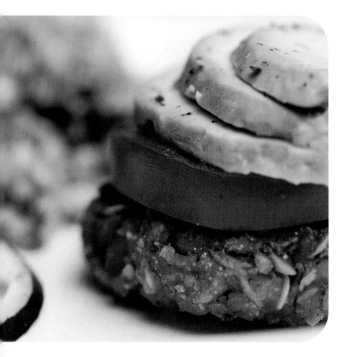

A while back, I went to hear Rip Esselstyn, ex-firefighter, Ironman triathlete, and creator of the *Engine 2 Diet* speak at a Whole Foods Market, and he brought up this same subject, that he always gets asked about where he gets his protein from. He commented that when people ask this, our response should be, "What are you doing to make sure you don't get too much protein?" I thought that was brilliant, because it really helps us to look deeper at our eating habits and beliefs.

Yes, we do need protein to build muscle and for our bodies to thrive. I've been a vegan/vegetarian for a very, very long time, and I've *never* had a protein deficiency, *ever*! I've had other small deficiencies, such as vitamin D, but this has nothing to do with not eating meat. If you are truly concerned that you will not get enough protein, I have offered options in this plan to add more plant-based proteins so that you can rest easy.

What Is SAP?

SAP, or sabotaging addictive patterns, are, in my opinion, the goo in our psychological self that holds us back from really getting and achieving what we want. How many times have you started a healthy eating regimen/diet only to fall off track three days later or completely sabotage yourself when you were done? How many times have you started a new project or even a relationship and noticed that old patterns arise that sabotage your efforts to really show up as your best self?

SAP, or sabotaging addictive patterns, are, in my opinion, the goo in our psychological self that holds us back from really getting and achieving what we want.

These patterns are what keep you from true success in many areas of your life. I will give you exercises each evening to complete during the 14 days that will help you take a deeper look at these patterns, as well as help you begin to shift them so that you don't have to keep coming up against them every time you start something new or challenging.

This will most likely be the hardest and most difficult part of this cleanse program. For many people, following a meal plan can be a simple task. It's the deeper work that people tend to shy away from, because it feels scary or too overwhelming. Believe me, I completely understand. I have been dealing with my own SAP all my life, and I am constantly working to shift it and be aware of it when it comes up. And it's so worth it when I truly overcome a SAP that has been running my life. It's what true freedom is all about.

The exercises I provide, called "Zap the SAP," will gently guide you to take a deeper look inside yourself. If you feel a tinge of fear, or want to throw it all in the bag as you read this, I encourage you to keep moving forward. Real change happens outside of your comfort zone.

And I get that change is scary for many, and even though you may want to grow as an individual, your subconscious mind can resist it on many levels. The resistance is at work inside

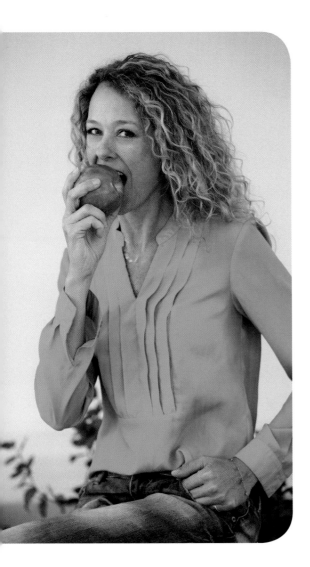

of you, without you even knowing it. You do what you know, until you know differently, and that is what this program is created to do: show you a different way of being, behaving, and reacting on every level—not only the physical but the mental and emotional as well.

What Can I Expect?

Cleansing can sometimes be an intense process depending on what your diet/life is like prior to beginning. I will give an overview here of some things you can expect while going through the process. It doesn't mean that you will feel all of these things, but you will most likely experience the detox "ickies" during the first three to five days of the program. The thing to remember is that the "negative" effects of detoxing are temporary, while the positive effects are more permanent, including the SAP you will be zapping.

It's hard for me to know exactly how your body will respond, as we are all different. Even if you drink five cups of coffee a day and eat sugar daily, you might not have the detox ickies as bad as someone who eats cleaner. It's all about metabolism, what is stored in your tissues, how you digest/assimilate nutrients, and so on.

Even people who eat a healthy diet can have a buildup in their system from environmental or even emotional toxins that haven't been cleared or dealt with. Stress is another huge form of toxicity in our body, especially when we don't manage it well. It can throw our bodies off in many ways and cause them to become overly acidic and ripe for disease.

There are so many factors to consider when it comes to your health, which is why I have included exercises that touch on the physical, mental, and emotional aspects of life. Here are some detox symptoms you may encounter during the first few days:

- Achy lower extremities and lower back

- Bloating and gas

- Cold and flu symptoms

- Constipation

- Emotional upset

- Fatigue/lethargy

- Headaches

- Skin eruptions

- Clogged or running sinuses

Remember, these symptoms are temporary and will be so worth the ride to your most optimal, healthy self. I always tell my clients that strong symptoms are good, even though they don't feel good, because it means that your body is actually purging the toxins and doing its job. And, you really get to feel the strong effects of these toxins you have been ingesting when they leave your body.

> Remember, these symptoms are temporary and will be so worth the ride to your most optimal, healthy self.

Again, keep in mind that everyone is different, and there is no way of knowing what your symptoms will be or how long they will last. The best thing you can do is to be prepared with a clear calendar and time to be able to rest and restore during the detox period. This is why it's imperative that you pick a time in your life when you know you can take care of you! You do not want to push your body when it's in detoxification mode. This will only put undue stress on your system, which will make it harder to clear toxins.

Here are some natural remedies for detox ickies, as described on previous page. If you get constipated, you want to be sure you nip this in the bud so that your body can expel any toxins as quickly as possible and you do not get backed up in the process.

Constipation:

- Drink plenty of water.

- Add 1 to 2 tablespoons ground flax seed to your salads or morning smoothie.

- Take magnesium citrate powder before bed each evening until relief.

- Take buffered vitamin C powder in your daily smoothie (2,000 mg).

Headaches:

- Stay well hydrated by drinking plenty of water.

- Massage peppermint essential oil on your temples
  (avoid getting it too close to your eyes).

- Keep a regular sleep schedule.

- Use a homeopathic "headache" remedy (such as Hylands).

- Drink AI Tea (see the recipe section under "Other Shakes, Teas, and Comfort Treats").

Bloating and Gas:

- Drink 1 tablespoon of apple cider vinegar in 10 ounces of water 20 minutes
  before meals.

- Use digestive enzymes; I like Ortho Digestzyme by Ortho Molecular Products
  (see resource section), but any digestive enzyme, including HCL, will work.

- Drink peppermint or ginger tea.

- Drink AI Tea (see the recipe section under "Other Shakes, Teas, and Comfort Treats").

Achy Joints/Back:

- Take an Epsom salts bath.

- Do some light stretching.

- Get a massage.

Flu-like Symptoms:

- Stay hydrated with plenty of water.

- Maintain a regular sleep schedule.

- Try a warm bath.

- Drink ginger tea or AI Tea (see the recipe section under "Other Shakes, Teas, and Comfort Treats").

Fatigue/Lethargy:

- Maintain a regular sleep schedule and take naps if you need to.

- Do some light exercise for at least 20 minutes to get your blood pumping. I know this may sound counterproductive, but this will be a chance to really tune in to your body and see what it needs.

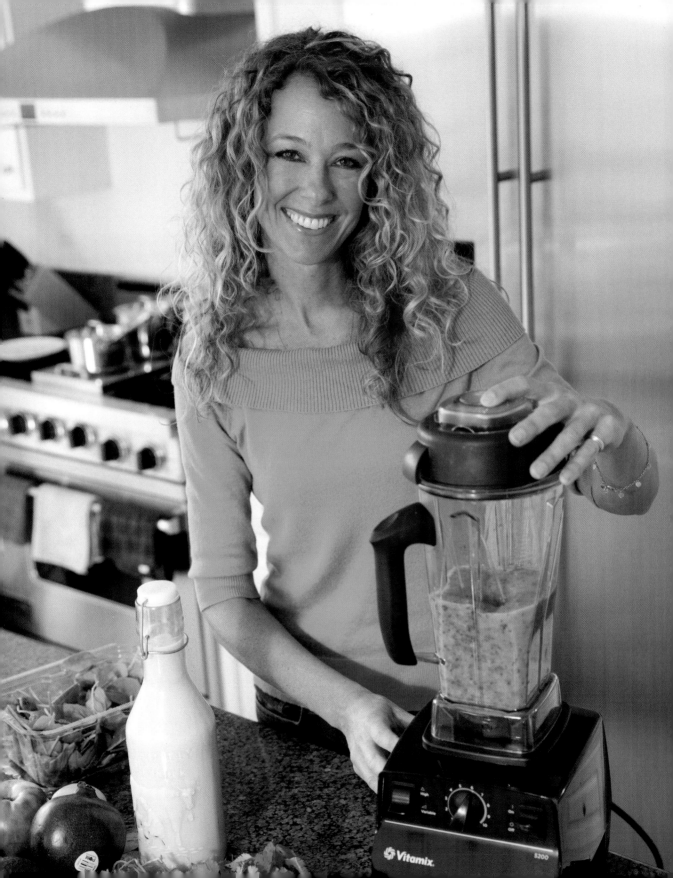

Chapter 4

Preparation Week

Now that I've given you all the ins and outs, and hopefully answered all your questions, I hope that you feel equipped to get going and start the Preparation Week. This week is all about getting yourself mentally, physically, and emotionally prepared to start the program. It's important that you read through all the steps in Preparation Week, and then schedule in certain items, like the "Kitchen Clear-Out." If you follow the ongoing steps I provide, you will experience the full benefit of this program. The more prepared you are, the better success you will have now, which will set you up for the long term as well. I want you to go into this feeling excited, ready, and self-assured.

I am guessing that if you were to make any other big decisions in your life, you would most likely have a plan. Well, this *is* a big decision you have made, so I am providing you with a plan on how to do it so that you will have the best, most rewarding experience, which will give you back your life. Remember, this is a lifelong journey. It doesn't end after these two weeks. So even though I have provided this plan, you will need to commit to yourself and this journey moving forward. When we are focusing on the prevention of illness and disease, we need consistency and commitment, two behaviors that will take you very far with anything in life, really.

Weaning: The Coffee and Sugar Smack Down

I always feel that going cold turkey is the most powerful when giving up any slow poison, but you have to find what is right for you. It may be hard to go cold turkey if you work a full-time job and need to function. Sometimes it's best to start this process on a weekend so that you can have the time/space to rest if you need to, and you don't have to be completely alert and coherent as you would at your job.

Giving up coffee and sugar may be the hardest part of this cleanse for most. When these substances leave our body, they usually tend to create upset in our system (as we learned in "What Can I Expect?" in Chapter 3). Below I have explained how you can cut back and wean yourself slowly, so that your body can acclimate more easily.

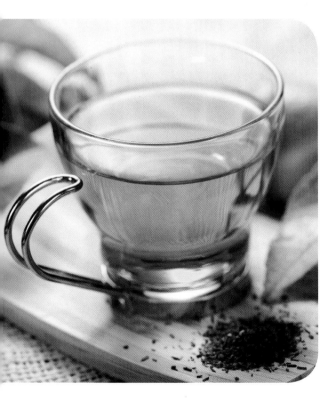

Coffee

Cut back to one-half regular and one-half decaf coffee for the first few days of the prep week. If you drink coffee in the afternoon, switch to green tea. If you drink multiple cups of coffee per day, make sure that every cup is made with one-half decaf.

You will eventually want to get off caffeine completely, and I understand that you may love the taste of coffee, so check out "Tea and Coffee Substitutes" in Chapter 7. By Day 5, you should only be drinking decaf and maybe one cup of green tea in the morning or afternoon. By Day 7, you want to be completely off any caffeine, including the green tea.

Sugar

This sweet, seductive poison always leaves you wanting more anytime you ingest it. Your body has become so addicted to it that you probably don't know what it feels like to live without it or how good you can feel without it. I always say, we don't know until we know. What most of my clients realize after going through my cleanses is that they didn't know they could feel as good as they do without sugar and coffee. Their addiction to these substances has them believing otherwise.

What most of my clients realize after going through my cleanses is that they didn't know they could feel as good as they do without sugar and coffee.

Sugar will be hard to give up because of its addictive nature. When you eat it, it releases serotonin in the brain, which is a feel-good chemical. This is temporary, of course, and you feel good for a short period of time, but it doesn't last. Over time it even depletes this very important neurotransmitter, which, in turn, can cause depression down the road.

Sometimes sugar detox effects are stronger than any others. Some of the things you may experience are headaches, dizziness, fatigue, and mood swings. I know this doesn't sound like much fun, but just remember *why* you are doing this, and that once you kick this very nasty habit, your life and your health will benefit more than you can ever imagine. Keep the bigger picture in sight, no matter what you do.

If you are a soda drinker, *stop* right now. There is no substitute for soda, as there is with coffee. Just *stop*. Trust me, this will benefit you more than you know. Soda is responsible for many adult diseases, which I have mentioned previously, like type-2 diabetes, obesity, and insulin resistance. Remember, we are learning how to eat and live preventatively.

If you do not drink soda, but you know you have a sugar addiction, spend this week cutting back tremendously so that you are sugar free by Day 1 of the program. You can use lower glycemic sweeteners during Prep Week (such as grade B maple syrup, coconut sugar, raw honey, or liquid stevia), but remember, sugar is sugar, and although all of it is not created equal, it still has the same effect on your body. You will want to cut back as much as you possibly can, even on the first day of Prep Week. Be very mindful of everything you put into your mouth.

You can do this by reading labels and staying away from any refined sugars that are on the "What to Avoid" list (see Chapter 5).

Don't worry, though. During this program you will be ingesting lower glycemic sugar (in the form of fruit) and complex carbohydrates, which also include fiber. Sugar is in many foods, including broccoli, but just know that when you are eating it in a natural form, it enters the body differently and processes differently, especially since the fiber is still in tact. We do need sugar to feed our muscles and our brains, especially after a workout, so you will be getting plenty of natural sugars to support this, but you'll be leaving a refined sugar addiction behind.

Giving Up Gluten

Gluten is challenging to let go of, not because of an addictive nature, but more because it's in almost everything! You will not be eating any processed foods during this cleanse, so it will be pretty easy to steer clear of it. As you do your "Kitchen Clear-Out," I suggest reading labels of any foods you have in your cabinet so that you can get an idea of how many foods do contain gluten (see "What to Avoid" in Chapter 5). It's often used as a filler in processed foods because it's cheap. To see a full up list of all ingredients that are often disguised as gluten, type abt.cm/MvxAeH in your web browser. Just like sugar, gluten can show up on labels as "fancy" names.

You will most likely not get any detox effects when giving up gluten, but what you will notice is how much better your digestion feels, and your energy may also soar as you rid your body of this sticky glue.

Most people aren't sure what gluten is and the effects it may have on the body, so I will explain it to you. There are also some amazing resources out there that talk more in-depth about the negative effects of it. One of those is the book called *Wheat Belly* written by Dr. William Davis. It's a really eye-opening read if you want to learn more about gluten. Gluten is basically the sticky protein found in wheat, barley, and rye. Most wheat products today have been so overly hybridized that our bodies do not know how to process them anymore. This is why kids today are riddled with allergies, and many people have gluten sensitivities or allergies. You may not be allergic to gluten, but it's very probable that you have a sensitivity to it. One way to find out is to eliminate it and see what changes you feel. You will also know more once you add it back in, if you decide to. Your body will usually respond immediately if you are sensitive to it. You could feel bloated, gassy, lethargic or you could have a headache with sinus issues. If this happens, you most likely have an allergy or sensitivity to it. Won't it feel good to really know for sure?

Most wheat products today have been so overly hybridized that our bodies do not know how to process them anymore. This is why kids today are riddled with allergies, and many people have gluten sensitivities or allergies.

I would suggest just cutting it out during Preparation Week if possible. If not and you want to finish up some foods you have in your house, that's fine. You get to choose how you want to do it, and what I find is that many people start to feel better almost immediately after giving it up, so why not go for it?

Alcohol and Animal Products

In "Getting Started: The Ins and Outs" in Chapter 1, I talked a lot about why it's important to give up alcohol and animal products. You can revisit that section, if you are unclear.

Again, going cold turkey with these two are best, but if you want to get your last couple drinks in the week prior, go for it. I always say that committing and just doing it is best, but again, you know yourself best, and you may want to have a little pre-cleanse party before going cold turkey. Just remember that every choice you make has a consequence, good or bad.

If you are accustomed to eating animal products every day at one of your meals, this may be a hard transition for you. I promise, you will not feel deprived, and by including tempeh in the meal plan, you will get to eat meals that at least resemble meat in texture. This whole cleanse is *only* 14 days, so you can go back to having meat afterward if your body wants it (I explain more about this in the final chapter of this book, "Post-Clean in 14 Transition Guidelines").

Prepping for Success: Kitchen Clear-Out

Clearing and cleaning out your kitchen is an important step to preparing yourself for this program. Go through your refrigerator and cabinets and toss any food that is processed or that contains refined sugar and preservatives. This will most likely be any food that comes in a bag, box, or can. Throw away any dried herbs and spices that are more than six months old. Spices lose their potency and flavor after this time period. Be sure to store them in a dark, cool, dry place, not over your heated stove.

You also want to be sure your refrigerator is clean and ready to be filled with lots of delicious, lush, fresh veggies. If you live with others in the household and they are not cleansing with you, make a special space for the foods you will be eating during the cleanse. Dedicate a shelf in your pantry and a drawer/spot in your fridge. This process will take anywhere from one to three hours depending on the state of your kitchen.

If you have bags of sugar in your cupboard for baking, save them to make body scrubs using coconut oil, jojoba oil, or almond oil to give away as gifts (it's easy: just mix two parts sugar to one part oil; add the oil from a few vitamin E capsules, and you're done).

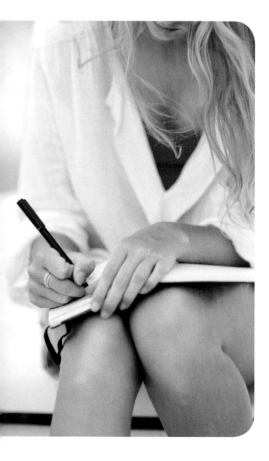

Journaling

Pick up a new journal to use during this program. You will want to actually put pen to paper instead of typing, because it is super powerful for the brain to connect with actual writing, to help clear habits. If you have never done any journaling, do not worry. I will explain more about it as we go along.

You will find journal assignments listed throughout the two-week program, so use your journal for these, and carry it with you throughout the day, so that it's available to you whenever you need to jot down notes, feelings, questions, and so on.

Your first step during Preparation Week is to fill out Your Big Fat Why by answering the questions in Chapter 5. You will want to reference this often to keep yourself accountable, and to find motivation when you need it.

Support

I have opened up a special online group on Facebook for those of you who want extra support, accountability, and who have questions. I find that when people are going through a program together with others, it is much easier for them. To join this group, type in the URL: on.fb.me/19Daltz

You will want to actually put pen to paper instead of typing, because it is super powerful for the brain to connect with actual writing, to help clear habits.

Also, I think it's wise to let the people closest to you in your life, those who you trust, know what you are doing, and ask for their support. You will definitely come up against people who are not supportive, and it's best that you avoid them during the program, or don't even let them know what you are up to.

You will know who will be and who won't be supportive of your journey, so choose wisely who you tell and ask for support from. This is a really good practice in learning how to ask for what you want, which may tend to be something we may not be good at or used to. It's so liberating to be able to do this; I know it has changed my life!

Remember, also, that living by example is the best way to educate others about what you are doing. No one wants to feel threatened or like they are being preached to. Your results will speak for themselves, and people will notice. If they are interested, they will ask, and if they are not, they won't. A lot of times others will want to know why you're so happy, your eyes are bright, and you seem so light. If they ask, tell them!

Shopping, Prep, and Cooking

Days 5–7 of Preparation Week can be used to shop and cook food based off the first four or five days of the meal plan/shopping list. Be sure you go over the shopping list and craft it based on how many you will be cooking for, as well as any ingredients you will need for the snacks you choose (see Chapter 7, "Cooking and Shopping Tips").

All the recipes include serving sizes, so make sure to pay attention to that. You can always repeat meals, if you are only preparing meals for yourself. I realize that I have included a lot of options here and it's a lot of food, so feel free to repeat and eat leftovers. As long as you are staying within the guidelines of the foods you *can* eat, you will stay on track.

You want to be sure you have food available at all times to grab and go. You also want to have your snacks prepared and take your food to work with you, even if you are going to be running errands in the car all day. Being prepared is *key* to your success on this cleanse—and even moving forward in life post-cleanse. It will ensure that you don't fall off the wagon.

Helpful Kitchen Tools

You don't have to go out and buy a whole new kitchen full of brand-new shiny appliances, but there definitely are a few tools that will make this journey much simpler. You don't have to get everything on this list, but make sure to have the basics on hand.

Basic Kitchen Tools

- Sharp chef's knife
- Large wooden or bamboo cutting board
- Blender: High-speed is best, like a Vitamix, but any blender will do
- Various wooden spoons
- Fine sieve strainer: inexpensive and a must in the kitchen for rinsing grains and beans
- Large soup pot
- Sauté pan with a lid or a wok

Other Helpful Items

- Food processor: great for making homemade hummus and lentil burgers
- Microplane: for grating ginger, garlic, nutmeg, and so on
- Lemon squeezer
- Rice cooker: make grains in a pinch without even paying attention

PREPARATION WEEK CHECKLIST

Daily ○ Cut back on coffee, sugar, and gluten (follow instructions given at the beginning of this chapter. By the end of Preparation Week you should be totally off coffee, sugar, and gluten).

○ Wean off animal products and alcohol.

Day 1 ○ Buy a journal.

○ Fill out Your Big Fat Why (see Chapter 5).

○ Join the Clean in 14 Facebook group at: on.fb.me/19Daltz

Day 2 ○ Read through Chapter 6, "Food Basics and the Meal Plans"

Day 3 ○ Clean out the refrigerator and cupboards of anything that is on the "What to Avoid" list in Chapter 5.

○ Check to be sure you are stocked with basic kitchen tools (see list on previous page).

Day 4 ○ Start to put together your shopping list based on your situation (see "Cooking and Shopping Tips" in Chapter 7).

Day 5 ○ Shop for the first four days of food.

Day 6 and 7 ○ Prep and cook meals for Days 1–4, including snacks.

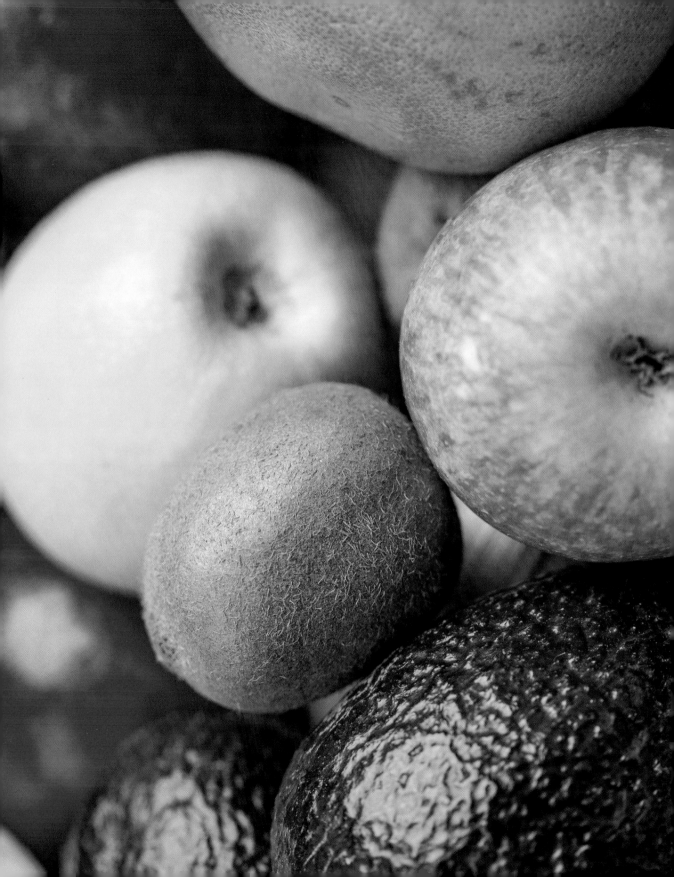

Chapter

5

Let's *Do* It!

Picking Your Start Date

The best thing to do is to choose a time when you know you do not have a lot going on, an upcoming vacation, or other huge commitments or social events on your calendar. Of course, life will always be life, and it will always be busy, so you can always find an excuse not to start.

You will know when the "right" time is. You will be ready. You will feel it. Chances are, you probably are ready, considering you bought this book. If you feel scared, that's a good sign. As I mentioned earlier, it means this is important to you. Nothing that's worth anything is ever easy, is it? There will be all kinds of ways your SAP will try to talk you out of beginning, so the best thing to do is pick a date and *do it*! Even better, get someone on board to do it with you! It's always more fun to have an accountability partner, and, of course, there is always the Clean in 14 support board on Facebook, so you can come there for any support you need too. It's best to clear your calendar as much as possible during this program. You will need time to rest more, do your exercises, and engage fully in the program. Starting the 14-day cleanse on a Monday is good because you will be ready to shop for the food, and batch cook over the weekend prior. However you choose to do it, be sure you open up the space for yourself. *You are worth it!*

I have given you a whole week of preparation so that you can be fully prepared and on track before starting the actual cleanse. The Prep Week is a *very* important part of this program and must be followed in order for you to be successful during this program, so if you skipped over that chapter, please go back and do it.

Make sure you set aside a full three weeks to integrate yourself into this process. You want to be fully present and committed and not go into it feeling ambivalent, even though there may be some fear present. You must know *why* you are doing this, and what you want to get out of it before you get started.

Your Big Fat Why

As I mentioned above, you must have a big enough why before you start this program. Having a big enough why will help keep you accountable to yourself. If you feel yourself slipping, you can always revisit your why to motivate you. I suggest hanging it somewhere in plain sight so that you can see it daily as you go through this process.

I am going to make it easy for you and give you a chance to really think about it and *write it down*. When we write down our intentions or "whys," it makes them stronger. They are a powerful tool to help hold you accountable and to show you why you are doing something.

Here are some questions to consider when thinking about your Big Fat Why:

- Am I willing to be uncomfortable and to move beyond my previous limitations to grow and change?

- What has held me back in the past from fully stepping into my truest, healthiest, and highest self?

- Am I willing to shift these behaviors and take contrary action (to do the opposite of what I have done before)?

- What will be different this time compared to others when I have let my SAPs seep in and ruin my efforts?

Now take out your journal and get busy. I promise this piece of action will be invaluable to your journey now, and moving forward.

The Health Scale: 1 to 10

When I think about my health and how important it is to me, I always use the 1 to 10 scale. I also use this scale with all my clients because it's super powerful in helping them to really see where they stand with their commitment to their journey.

I ask, "On a scale of one to ten, with one being the least and ten being the most, how important is your health?" Ninety-nine percent of the time my clients will answer "ten." I do have a few that will say "seven" or "eight" because of their fear of missing out, or they think that if they are super healthy, they can never have sugar or chocolate again and they will be missing out on life, not living, in a sense. I can totally appreciate this honesty, and being healthy doesn't have to mean missing out or feeling deprived; in fact, I feel it's just the opposite. I focus on all the foods I can enjoy and all that is available to me, and believe me, there's a lot!

There is always a healthier version available for your favorite food. Granted, it may not taste exactly the same, but as you get healthier and cleaner, your body will actually crave the healthier version. More often than not, when I have clients dip back into their old ways of eating, they do not enjoy it anymore, and they love how they feel when they are eating clean. They now prefer the healthy version, and the amazing flavor and health benefits it offers.

The body starts to change internally; it no longer wants the unhealthy stuff. It starts to crave the good stuff. In a way, this process pushes out the bad to make room for the good. Your taste buds will even change and food will have more flavor.

The body starts to change internally; it no longer wants the unhealthy stuff. It starts to crave the good stuff. In a way, this process pushes out the bad to make room for the good. Your taste buds will even change and food will have more flavor.

The Three W's, and I Don't Mean the Worldwide Web

The 3 W's—Why you eat, When you eat, and What you eat—will be *huge* for you during these 14 days. Asking yourself these three simple questions every time you reach for food will give you huge insight into your daily habits.

You will begin to see that you might eat when you're not hungry. Or you may eat to comfort yourself. Or you may overeat when you are uncomfortable in a social situation. Or you may choose food that is not so healthy for you because you are in a rush or don't feel like dealing. You may choose convenience over health, or you might turn to food as an emotional crutch. Whatever your habits are, these three quick questions will help you on your journey to breaking them down, step-by-step. Let's look a little deeper.

Why You Eat

Why do we eat? Well, because we need food to survive and to fuel our bodies. Yet all too often, people do not eat for this reason. They eat for many other reasons, including connection, comfort, to feel love or social acceptance, to feed some emotion or pattern, or because it's noon on the clock, or dinnertime. Too often we don't tune in to the needs of our body and what it wants. Our society has become so toxically overloaded and poisoned by processed foods, sugar, alcohol, caffeine, and gluten that our bodies can no longer tell what they need. We eat to feed an addiction or a bad habit.

In this process you will learn more about eating when your body gives you cues. As you become cleaner, your body will want cleaner foods. The so-called bad foods/toxins will be pushed out and your body will start to crave healthful, whole foods, like on the menu I have provided. You will learn to eat to fuel your body, to give it energy, and to feed it nutrients that it may not have been getting prior to this program. Your "why" of eating will change drastically as you go through the 14-day cleanse.

When You Eat

The when and why of eating really do go hand in hand. Anytime you put food in your mouth, it's important to first ask yourself if you are really hungry or if you are just giving in to a craving. Notice your eating patterns throughout the day. Do you skip meals? Do you eat sporadically? Can you even tune in to your body and decipher what hunger truly feels like? Do you have a consistent eating schedule? Or do you just eat when you are hungry, listening to your body's cues? All of these questions will give you insight into when you eat, and if the timing of your meals is benefiting you or overfeeding you.

The when and why of eating really do go hand in hand. Anytime you put food in your mouth, it's important to first ask yourself if you are really hungry or if you are just giving in to a craving.

What You Eat

During this cleanse, you will know what to eat, but what about in your day-to-day life before you embarked on this journey? Did you pay attention to what you ate? Did you just grab whatever was easy and convenient, even if it wasn't healthy? How much processed food did you eat? How much sugar? Remember that 1 to 10 scale I explained earlier? Well, I want you to also use that scale when you put food into your mouth, and give each food a score from 1 to 10 on where it lives on that scale.

You want to eat foods that are on the upper end of the scale, landing in the 8 to 10 region. This includes whole foods, grains, beans, veggies, fruits, nuts, seeds, lean proteins, and so on. Other foods, such as fast food, pastries, and sugar-laden foods, would be in the 1 to 2 range on the scale. As you go through this cleanse, you will be putting plenty of 8, 9, and 10 foods in your mouth. When you complete the program, you'll really want to pay attention to where the food you are eating ranges on that scale.

I am not saying you always have to eat in the 8 to 10 range. Maybe sometimes you will dip into the below 5 range, but keep in mind that there are always good or bad consequences to the choices we make in life, no matter what they are. We are a product or consequence of every choice we have made in our lives up until now, and will continue to be thereafter. This is a powerful way to see life.

What's In and What's Out

Below are basic reference lists of "What to Avoid" and "What to Enjoy" during the next 14 days—and hopefully beyond that.

If it helps, scan a copy of the lists or take a photo with your phone and keep it with you at all times so you are never at a loss for what you can and can't have during this process. Make sure you become very familiar with these lists. The basic rule of thumb is to not ingest any processed foods and to stay away from those foods and beverages outlined in "What to Avoid" below. I know this list may seem extensive, but this is because there are so many hidden ingredients in foods that I want to be sure you are educated for the long term as well.

What to **AVOID**

Be sure to always read labels when buying anything. Even condiments and canned beans can have added sugar or preservatives.

- Alcohol
- Animal products: meat, poultry, fish, and eggs
- Artificial sweeteners, including gum, mints, diet soda and drinks, and so on
- Caffeinated beverages: green tea, yerba maté, white tea, coffee, black tea, and decaf coffees and teas
- Chocolate, raw cacao, or cocoa
- Condiments sweetened with high fructose corn syrup or sugar: ketchup, salad dressings, mustard, and so on (read labels)
- Dairy products: cheese, yogurt, and milk
- Fried foods
- Fruit juices: bottled juices, including Naked Juice (except pure cranberry and pure pomegranate juice, not from concentrate)
- Grains/gluten: wheat, rye, barley, couscous, spelt, farro
- Non-vegan protein powders and casein/whey
- Over-the-counter medications (if possible)
- Processed foods (Foods that contain chemicals, preservatives, additives and ingredients you can't pronounce) exceptions include nut milks, beans, tempeh, and certain gluten-free grains

- Refined sugars: dextrose, maltose, sucralose, cane sugar, high fructose corn syrup (HFCS), evaporated cane juice, raw cane sugar, dried cane syrup

- Soda (including those sweetened with artificial sweeteners)

- Unfermented soy products that are overly processed (tempeh, Bragg's aminos and miso are okay)

- White potatoes, white flour/bread, and white rice

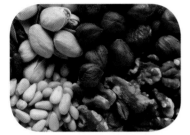

What to **ENJOY**

- Nut, seed, and gluten-free grain milks (unsweetened)

- Beans/legumes: dried or canned are okay (drain and rinse thoroughly)

- Coconut milk and coconut water

- Raw nut and seed crackers such as flax, almond, pumpkin seed, etc.

- Fruits: all (except dried and store-bought fruit juices)

- Herbal teas including roasted dandelion root tea (purchase at any health food store or online. My favorite is Traditional Medicinals)

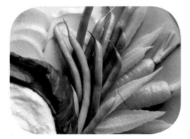

- Juice: pure cranberry and pure pomegranate juice, not from concentrate

- Nuts and seeds: raw only

- Nut butters (unsweetened)

- Coffee substitutes: Teeccino, Dandy Blend

- Tempeh and miso

- Veggies: all, and vegan protein powders (see Resources section)

- Water—plenty of it—and hot lemon water each morning (see page 25)

- Whole grains: amaranth, buckwheat, millet, oats (make sure they're not processed where wheat is processed), quinoa, sorghum, teff, and brown or wild rice

Besides avoiding the food and beverages listed above, you also need to avoid calorie counting, weighing yourself daily, and unsupportive people, all of which could take your focus off the reason you've embarked on this journey. See "A Word About Portions," in Chapter 6. Remember, this program is about learning a whole new way of eating and living, not just about losing weight. It's about learning to avoid the CRAP and the SAPs that are preventing you from living your best life.

During the two weeks of the program, besides enjoying the new foods and recipes, and getting creative in the kitchen, you'll also enjoy seeing and feeling the changes in your body (even the subtle ones). Be sure to enjoy some type of daily physical exercise as you go through the program, as this will enhance the effects of the cleanse.

CHEAT SHEET • ENJOY

- ✓ Veggies, Fruits, Whole Grains, Legumes, Nuts, and Seeds
- ✓ Being Creative in the Kitchen
- ✓ Daily Exercise
- ✓ Plenty of Water and Herbal Tea
- ✓ Living by Example
- ✓ Seeing and Feeling the Changes in Your Body
- ✓ Knowing You Are Doing Something Positive for *You!*

Chapter

6

Food Basics and the Meal Plans

A s you will notice, I use a lot of the same ingredients in different dishes. I've chosen specific ingredients that will not only help your body detoxify and cleanse itself but that are also loaded with nutrients and protein. The ingredients in the recipes are all easy to find in most grocery stores, but I have also included a resource section in the back so you can order some things online, like roasted dandelion root tea and protein powder.

All of the dishes are crafted with health *and* flavor combined—something people don't always think about when they hear that a particular food is healthy. They usually think it will be tasteless.

Almost all of the salads can be eaten as meals, and I have repeated some of the meals so that any leftovers can be used as snacks or for the next day as per the meal plan, especially if you are the only one participating in the program. If you have a family, you may want to double some of the recipes. Many of my clients get their families to come on board, not by bribing them but by cooking the delicious food that is provided in the program, and by also living as an example. Most people cannot resist the amazing aromas coming from the kitchen, and the cool thing is that everyone benefits, whether they are cleansing or not.

The bowls served at both lunch and dinner are a great way to get a very filling meal in one easy dish by combining high-nutrient grains, beans, and veggies. Again, bowls are a great way to utilize any leftovers you may have on hand before you go shopping again, or cook more food.

Batch Cooking

Batch cooking is going to be your friend and a *huge* key to your success during these next 14 days. What I mean by this is that you spend a few blocked-out hours in the kitchen and prepare four days' worth of meals at a time. I have set up Days 5–7 of Preparation Week to be the days you shop, cook, and batch cook for the first actual week of the program. I also suggest you cook a pot of rice, quinoa, and lentils to have handy at all times to throw in salads, eat in a bowl with other veggies, and so on.

Peruse the recipes and see which items are used more than once that you can cook batches of, or precut veggies for certain dishes and snacks. For example, if a recipe calls for half a head of cauliflower, cut the whole thing up and store what you don't use in the recipe in the refrigerator to use in another recipe or snacking. I've done my best to group a lot of the ingredients together by days so that you can do this. Precutting all your veggies will also save you a lot of time, and it's always fun to put on some music and chop away while singing some tunes. I put all of my cut veggies in glass bowls as I cut them, so I can see all my hard work—and the beautiful colors—in front of me.

A Word about Portions

If you've read my first book, *The Karma Chow Ultimate Cookbook*, you will know that I am not a fan of calorie counting or weighing and measuring food. So you may be wondering, *How much exactly do I eat?* As you will notice, all of the recipes are broken into servings, but I did not include any calorie counts or nutritional information. I did this for a reason. I don't want you to worry about counting calories. These foods are high-nutrient, whole foods that are meant to support your body's natural detox ability. Calorie counting can oftentimes disconnect you from your food, and from listening to your body's own natural hunger cues. As I've mentioned before, the cleaner you eat, the better your body will be able to tell you what it needs.

I want you to really tune in now. Be present when you eat. Practice conscious eating (the Sixth Basic Principle given in Chapter 2). Give thanks for the amazing nourishment you are putting into your body. You spent all the time to cook it, so why not sit, relax, breathe, chew your food, and really enjoy it? I know this may sound a bit crazy, but trust me, your body knows. It will never betray you; it will only respond to the choices you make for it, and you are a product of all of your choices up until now. There are consequences to every choice you make, whether it's "good" or "bad." Yes, I know I keep repeating this, but it is true.

Start with a smaller portion, wait about 15 to 20 minutes, and then go back for more if you still feel hungry. I always eat out of a small-sized bowl versus a large plate. I then refill it if I need to, but usually a small portion is enough. Our culture has become accustomed to over-eating and not tuning in to the needs of our bodies, and that's why obesity and heart disease are growing at astronomical rates and people are suffering from ill health. Remember, this is a process. There is a learning curve. Your body has not been treated very well, and it will take time to change this, so be patient and consistent, and it will definitely begin to pay off.

If you find yourself hungry, please feel free to eat a snack either midmorning or mid-afternoon. You can have any leftovers as a snack, or any of the snacks listed on the snack list on page 74.

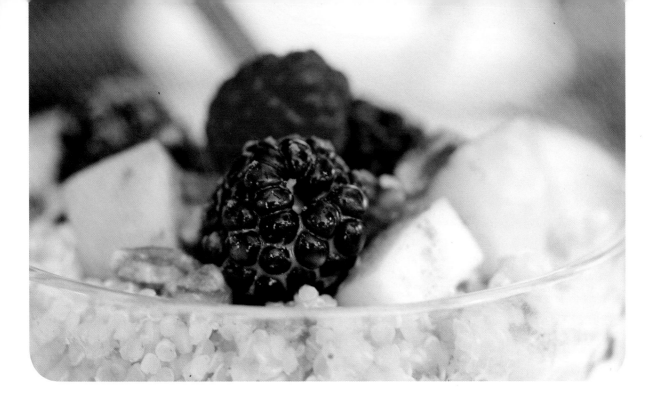

Day 1

Rising	○	Hot lemon water, (p. 25)
Breakfast	○	Power Protein Breakfast Bowl, (p.119)
Lunch	○	Kale and Quinoa Power Salad, (p. 147)
Post-Lunch Detoxifier (between 2:00 to 3:00 PM)	○	Roasted dandelion root tea
Dinner	○	Maple-Glazed Baked Tempeh, (p. 191), and Chopped Salad with Shallot Vinaigrette, (p. 149)
Pre-Sleep Elixir (optional)	○	Choice of AI Tea, (p. 139), Creamy Golden Milk, (p. 141), or herbal tea

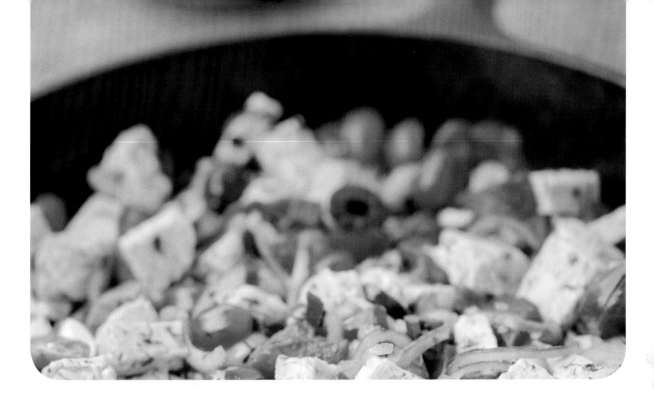

Day 2

Rising	○ Hot lemon water, (p. 25)
Breakfast	○ Mediterranean Veggie Scramble, (p. 121)
Lunch	○ Chopped Salad, (p. 149), with Sweet Pea Soup, (p. 177), and a scoop of quinoa
Post-Lunch Detoxifier (between 2:00 to 3:00 PM)	○ Roasted dandelion root tea
Dinner	○ Portobello Stacker with Chipotle Cashew Cheese, (p. 193), and Kale and Quinoa Power Salad, (p. 147)
Pre-Sleep Elixir (optional)	○ Choice of AI Tea, (p. 139), Creamy Golden Milk, (p. 141), or herbal tea

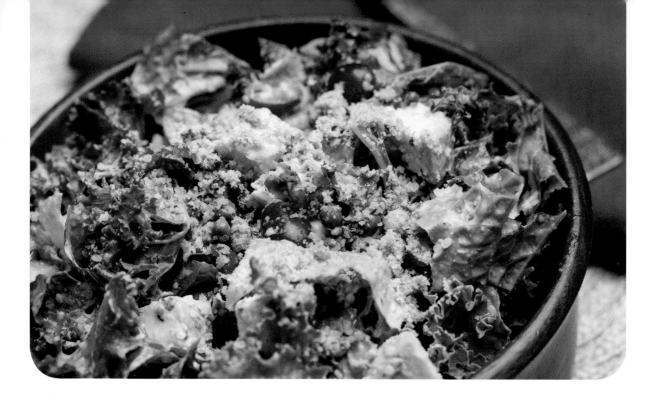

Day 3

Rising	○ Hot lemon water, (p. 25)
Breakfast	○ Fruit Bowl with Crème Sauce, (p. 123), or Green with Envy Smoothie, (p. 127)
Lunch	○ Creamy Kale and Avocado Caesar, (p. 155)
Post-Lunch Detoxifier (between 2:00 to 3:00 PM)	○ Roasted dandelion root tea
Dinner	○ Sweet Pea Soup, (p. 177), and Sweet and Savory Tempeh Tacos, (p. 199)
Pre-Sleep Elixir (optional)	○ Choice of AI Tea, (p. 139), Creamy Golden Milk, (p. 141), or herbal tea

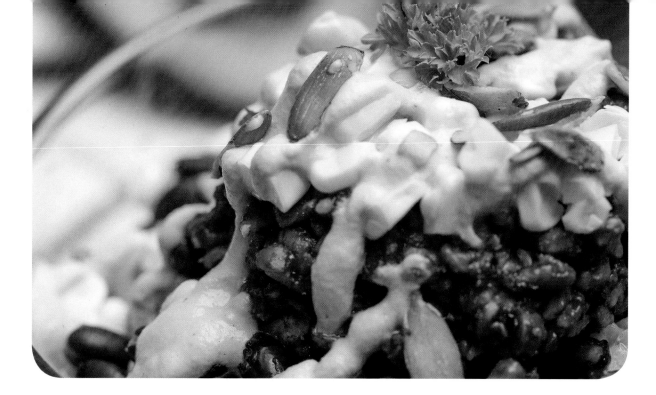

Day 4

Rising	○	Hot lemon water, (p. 25)
Breakfast	○	Ruby's Raspberry Dazzle Protein Shake, (p. 125)
Lunch	○	Taco Salad Bowl with Smoky Chipotle Dressing, (p. 201)
Post-Lunch Detoxifier (between 2:00 to 3:00 PM)	○	Roasted dandelion root tea
Dinner	○	Coconut Basil Stir-Fry, (p. 203), over quinoa with Creamy Kale and Avocado Caesar, (p. 155)
Pre-Sleep Elixir (optional)	○	Choice of AI Tea, (p. 139), Creamy Golden Milk, (p. 141), or herbal tea

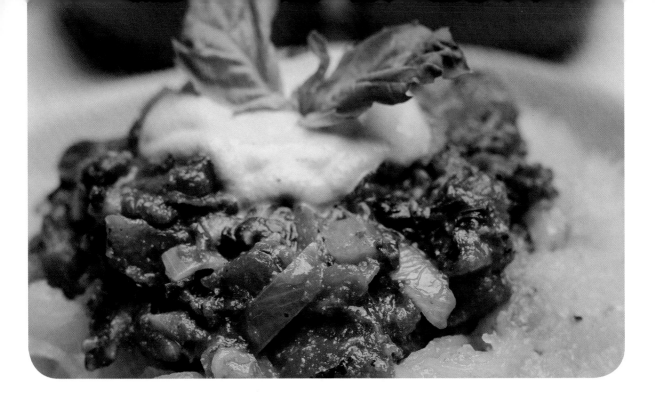

Day 5

Rising	○ Hot lemon water, (p. 25)
Breakfast	○ Power Protein Breakfast Bowl, (p. 119)
Lunch	○ Gracious Greek Salad, (p. 153), and Caribbean Black Bean Soup, (p. 179)
Post-Lunch Detoxifier (between 2:00 to 3:00 PM)	○ Roasted dandelion root tea
Dinner	○ Spaghetti Squash Italiano, (p. 205), with Herbed Brown Rice and Lentil Salad, (p. 151)
Pre-Sleep Elixir (optional)	○ Choice of AI Tea, (p. 139), Creamy Golden Milk, (p. 141), or herbal tea

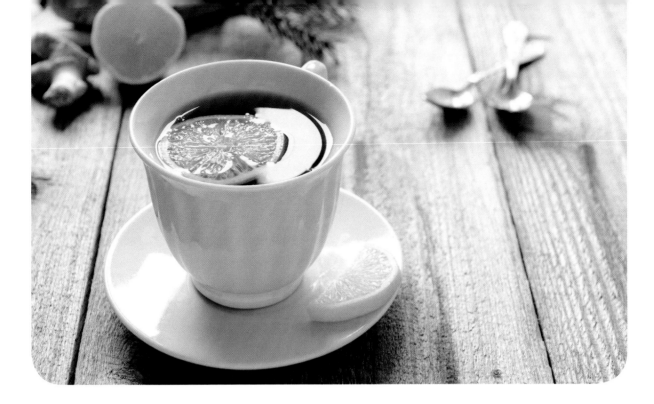

Day 6

Rising	○ Hot lemon water, (p. 25)
Breakfast	○ Green with Envy Smoothie, (p. 127)
Lunch	○ Spaghetti Squash Surprise Bowl, (p. 206)
Post-Lunch Detoxifier (between 2:00 to 3:00 PM)	○ Roasted dandelion root tea
Dinner	○ Curried Red Lentil Walnut Burger, (p. 209), and Snappy Slaw, (p. 157)
Pre-Sleep Elixir (optional)	○ Choice of AI Tea, (p. 139), Creamy Golden Milk, (p. 141), or herbal tea

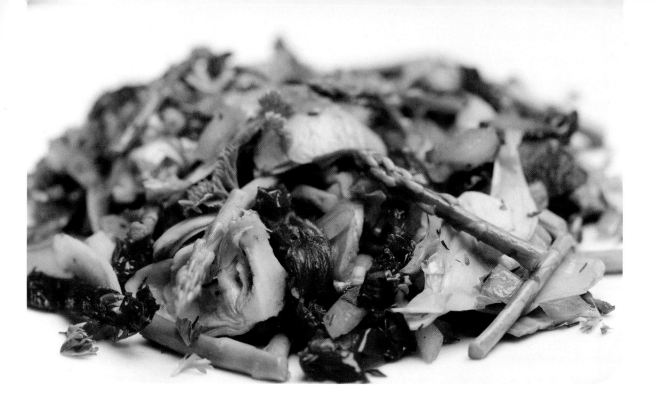

Day 7

Rising	○	Hot lemon water, (p. 25)
Breakfast	○	Gingery Miso Soup, (p. 130), with scoop of quinoa and avocado slices
Lunch	○	Curried Red Lentil Walnut Burger, (p. 209), on greens with Caribbean Black Bean Soup, (p. 179)
Post-Lunch Detoxifier (between 2:00 to 3:00 PM)	○	Roasted dandelion root tea
Dinner	○	Karma Chili Bowl, (p. 214), with Warmed Wild Mushroom and Asparagus Salad, (p. 169)
Pre-Sleep Elixir (optional)	○	Choice of AI Tea, (p. 139), Creamy Golden Milk, (p. 141), or herbal tea

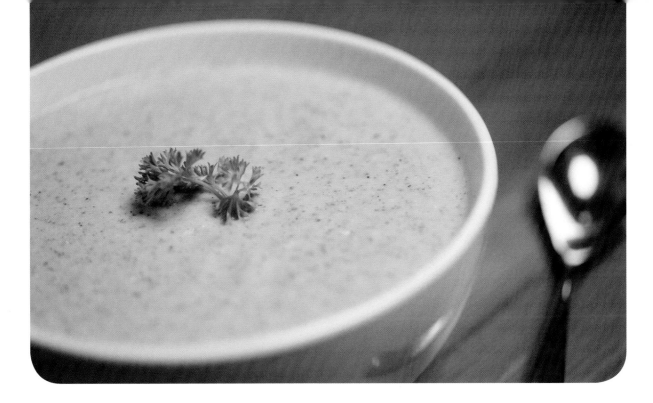

Day 8

Rising	○	Hot lemon water, (p. 25)
Breakfast	○	Fruit Bowl with Crème Sauce, (p. 123)
Lunch	○	Karma Chili Bowl, (p. 214), and Snappy Slaw, (p. 157)
Post-Lunch Detoxifier (between 2:00 to 3:00 PM)	○	Roasted dandelion root tea
Dinner	○	Gregarious Green Soup, (p. 181), and Indian Spiced Baked Yam, (p. 207)
Pre-Sleep Elixir (optional)	○	Choice of AI Tea, (p. 139), Creamy Golden Milk, (p. 141), or herbal tea

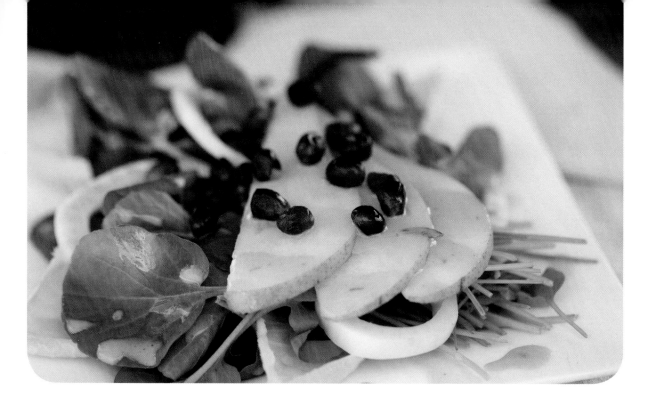

Day 9

Rising	○ Hot lemon water, (p. 25)
Breakfast	○ Green with Envy Smoothie, (p. 127)
Lunch	○ Watercress, Pear, and Fennel Salad, (p. 159), with Gregarious Green Soup, (p. 181)
Post-Lunch Detoxifier (between 2:00 to 3:00 PM)	○ Roasted dandelion root tea
Dinner	○ Mashed Basil Cauliflower "Potatoes", (p. 213), with Asian-Style Quinoa Salad, (p. 161)
Pre-Sleep Elixir (optional)	○ Choice of AI Tea, (p. 139), Creamy Golden Milk, (p. 141), or herbal tea

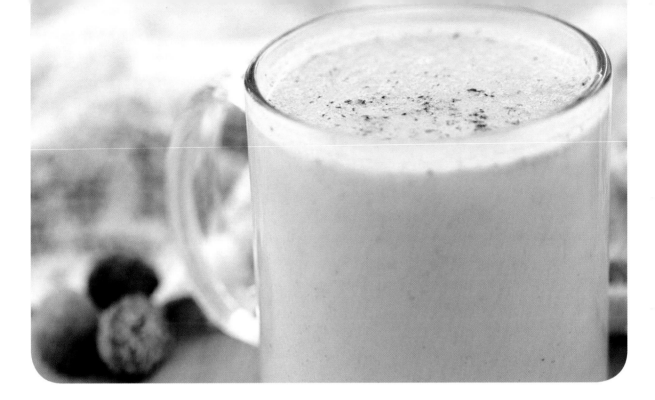

Day 10

Rising	○	Hot lemon water, (p. 25)
Breakfast	○	Energy Chia Breakfast Pudding, (p. 129), with fresh fruit
Lunch	○	Creamy Cauliflower Soup, (p. 187), with Asian-Style Quinoa Salad, (p. 161)
Post-Lunch Detoxifier (between 2:00 to 3:00 PM)	○	Roasted dandelion root tea
Dinner	○	Mexican Spiced Black Bean and Yam Bowl, (p. 215)
Pre-Sleep Elixir (optional)	○	Choice of AI Tea, (p. 139), Creamy Golden Milk, (p. 141), or herbal tea

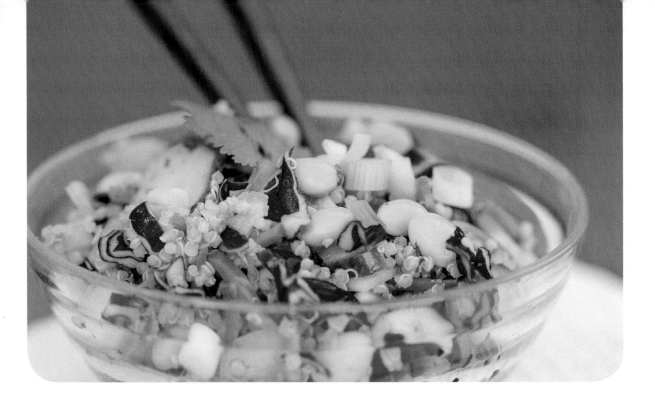

Day 11

Rising	○	Hot lemon water, (p. 25)
Breakfast	○	Savory Brekkie Bowl, (p. 131)
Lunch	○	Gregarious Green Soup, (p. 181), and a leafy green salad of your choice (see "Salad of Your Choice" p. 171 in the recipe section for ingredient ideas)
Post-Lunch Detoxifier (between 2:00 to 3:00 PM)	○	Roasted dandelion root tea
Dinner	○	Red Lentil Curry Stew, (p. 185), served over brown rice with Thai Cucumber Salad, (p. 165)
Pre-Sleep Elixir (optional)	○	Choice of AI Tea, (p. 139), Creamy Golden Milk, (p. 141), or herbal tea

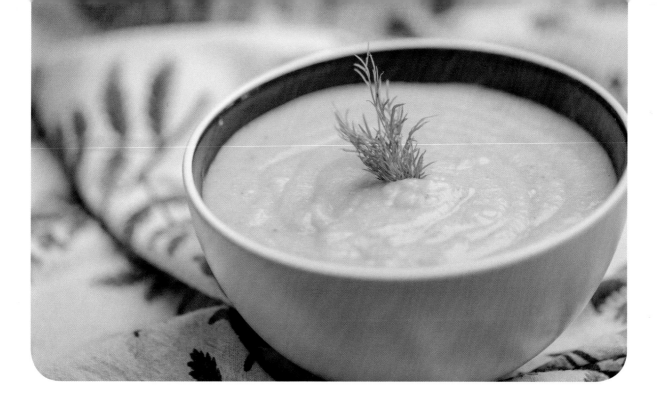

Day 12

Rising	○ Hot lemon water, (p. 25)
Breakfast	○ Ruby's Raspberry Dazzle Protein Shake, (p. 125)
Lunch	○ Creamy Cauliflower Soup, (p. 187), and Thai Cucumber Salad, (p. 165)
Post-Lunch Detoxifier (between 2:00 to 3:00 PM)	○ Roasted dandelion root tea
Dinner	○ Veggie Fajita Wraps, (p. 197), with White Bean and Thyme Soup, (p. 183)
Pre-Sleep Elixir (optional)	○ Choice of AI Tea, (p. 139), Creamy Golden Milk, (p. 141), or herbal tea

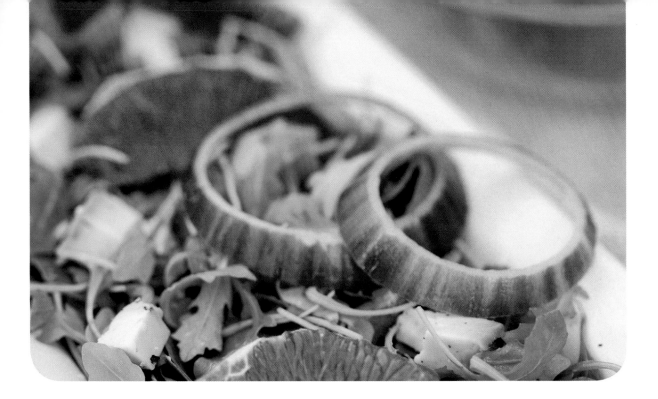

Day 13

Rising	○ Hot lemon water, (p. 25)
Breakfast	○ Energy Chia Breakfast Pudding, (p. 129)
Lunch	○ Red Lentil Curry Stew, (p. 185), with a leafy green salad of your choice (see "Salad of Your Choice" p. 171 in the recipe section)
Post-Lunch Detoxifier (between 2:00 to 3:00 PM)	○ Roasted dandelion root tea
Dinner	○ Grapefruit, Avocado, and Arugula Salad, (p. 163), with Roasted Root Veggies, (p. 217)
Pre-Sleep Elixir (optional)	○ Choice of AI Tea, (p. 139), Creamy Golden Milk, (p. 141), or herbal tea

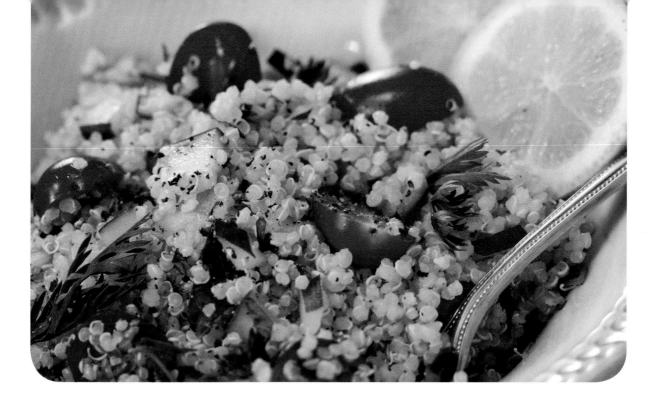

Day 14

Rising	○ Hot lemon water, (p. 25)
Breakfast	○ White Bean and Thyme Soup, (p. 183), with quinoa and avocado slices
Lunch	○ Roasted Root Veggies, (p. 217), with a leafy green salad of your choice (see "Salad of Your Choice" p. 171 in the recipe section)
Post-Lunch Detoxifier (between 2:00 to 3:00 PM)	○ Roasted dandelion root tea
Dinner	○ Quinoa Tabbouleh Salad, (p. 167), with Spicy Home-Style Collards, (p. 219)
Pre-Sleep Elixir (optional)	○ Choice of AI Tea, (p. 139), Creamy Golden Milk, (p. 141), or herbal tea

(see "Breakfast and Shakes" in the recipe section)

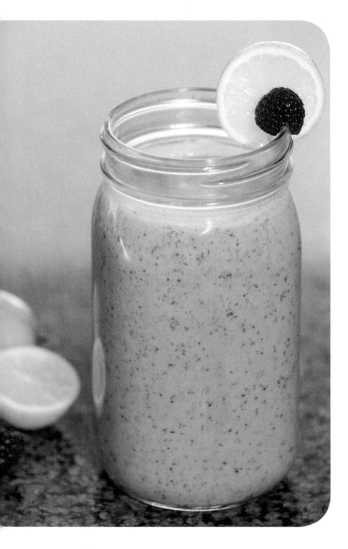

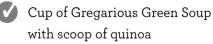 Energy Chia Breakfast Pudding (see "Breakfast and Shakes" in the recipe section)

Raw veggies and hummus/guacamole/bean dip

Piece of fruit with nuts or nut butter

Cup of Gregarious Green Soup with scoop of quinoa

Cup of rice with one-eighth avocado

Protein shake/smoothie or vegetable juice

Any of the other shakes or teas given in the recipe section

Raw flax crackers with hummus or guacamole

Any leftovers

Cooking and Shopping Tips

Prep Your Pantry

Hopefully, if you've been following the plan exactly, you have already cleaned out your pantry during Preparation Week. I also want you to go through it again before starting and see what foods you already have on hand that are part of the Clean in 14 recipes (spices, condiments, grains, oils, etc.). Use the shopping list starting on page 77 to help you. This will ensure that you don't overbuy and waste money.

Shop Only for the First Four Days' Worth of Food—Plan, Plan, Plan!

I know you are excited and ready to get started, but do not go out and buy everything to make meals for the entire 14 days. I have provided a shopping list for the first week of the program, but always *reassess* and buy what you need based on leftovers and unused food. Quantities *will vary*, so double-check recipes and use your discretion when shopping (if you are only shopping for one, buy less!). Your first shop will most likely be the most expensive because you are stocking up on the basics. Remember, a lot of the condiments you buy will last you a long time and can be used to keep your healthy lifestyle going after the cleanse. Be sure to stock up on herbal teas as well.

Ask for What You Need

You may have not heard of a lot of these foods before, so this is the perfect time to ask for help. When you get to the grocery store, find a friendly worker and ask them to help you. Most grocery store workers are more than happy to show you where specific foods are. This will be great practice for you and goes right along with your Action Items on Day 7 of the cleanse.

Batch Cooking Is Your Friend

Yes, I've already explained this earlier, but I really want you to know the importance of it and how it will help your success on the cleanse. Cook your food in batches for three to four days' worth of eating. Spend three to four hours on Saturday or Sunday the weekend prior to your start date to do your planning, shopping, chopping, and cooking all in one day. Schedule this in and make time!

Clean Your Greens

It's important to clean your greens as soon as you return home from shopping. This will ensure that your greens stay fresh. Wash them really well, spin them in a salad spinner, or drain them well, and store them in an airtight bag or container with a damp paper towel on top. This will keep your greens from wilting and losing nutritive value.

Buy Organic and Seasonal

Do your best to buy all organic veggies and fruits without thick skins. Also, if possible, buy fruit that is in season. You can substitute what you need to, depending on what's available in your area. To see a more comprehensive list of what you should try to buy organic, check out the resource section in the back.

Substitutes

If you cannot find certain greens or ingredients, or you don't like certain foods, you can substitute something else or leave them out. These recipes were created with foods that will help you to detox, but if you cannot stand something, I do not want you to suffer through it. Use your discretion.

Shopping List: Days 1 to 4

Veggies:
- ❏ 1 bag arugula
- ❏ 1 bok choy
- ❏ 1 head broccoli
- ❏ 1 bunch carrots
- ❏ 2 baskets cherry tomatoes
- ❏ 2 heads curly kale
- ❏ 2 endive
- ❏ 2 bulbs garlic
- ❏ 2-inch piece ginger
- ❏ 1 leek
- ❏ 1 10-ounce bag frozen peas
- ❏ 2 portobello mushrooms
- ❏ 2 red bell peppers
- ❏ 2 red onions
- ❏ 1 small head radicchio
- ❏ 1 head romaine
- ❏ 1 bunch scallions
- ❏ 1 shallot
- ❏ 1 small package white mushrooms
- ❏ 1 large zucchini

Fresh Herbs:
- ❏ Basil, 1 bunch
- ❏ 1 package fresh mint
- ❏ Rosemary, 1 bundle

Fruits:
- ❏ Fruits *(enough for smoothies, snacks, and fruit breakfast bowls)*
- ❏ 4–6 bananas *(freeze 3 in halves for smoothies)*
- ❏ 2 green apples
- ❏ 1 bag dates
- ❏ Fruit of choice for Fruit Bowl with Crème Sauce *(see recipe section)*
- ❏ 1 bag frozen raspberries *(10 ounces)*
- ❏ 1 bag frozen strawberries *(10 ounces)*
- ❏ 2 avocados
- ❏ 6 medium lemons
- ❏ 3 medium limes

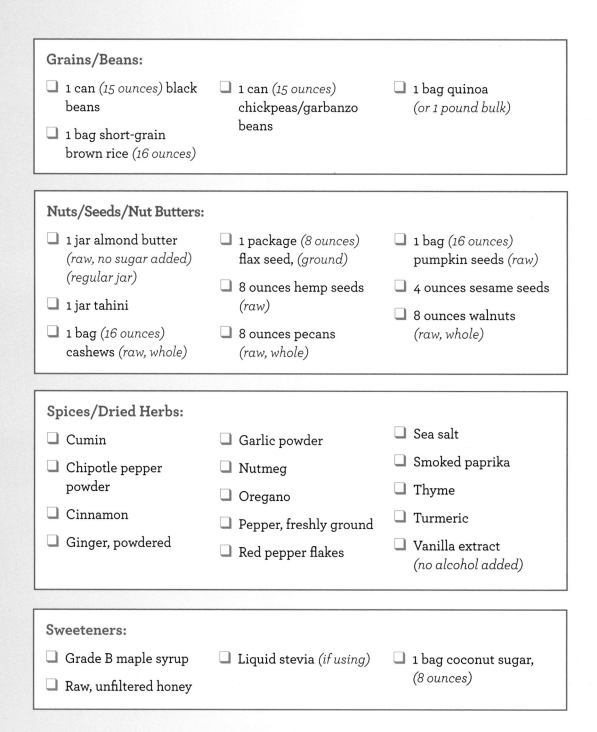

Grains/Beans:

- ☐ 1 can *(15 ounces)* black beans
- ☐ 1 bag short-grain brown rice *(16 ounces)*
- ☐ 1 can *(15 ounces)* chickpeas/garbanzo beans
- ☐ 1 bag quinoa *(or 1 pound bulk)*

Nuts/Seeds/Nut Butters:

- ☐ 1 jar almond butter *(raw, no sugar added) (regular jar)*
- ☐ 1 jar tahini
- ☐ 1 bag *(16 ounces)* cashews *(raw, whole)*
- ☐ 1 package *(8 ounces)* flax seed, *(ground)*
- ☐ 8 ounces hemp seeds *(raw)*
- ☐ 8 ounces pecans *(raw, whole)*
- ☐ 1 bag *(16 ounces)* pumpkin seeds *(raw)*
- ☐ 4 ounces sesame seeds
- ☐ 8 ounces walnuts *(raw, whole)*

Spices/Dried Herbs:

- ☐ Cumin
- ☐ Chipotle pepper powder
- ☐ Cinnamon
- ☐ Ginger, powdered
- ☐ Garlic powder
- ☐ Nutmeg
- ☐ Oregano
- ☐ Pepper, freshly ground
- ☐ Red pepper flakes
- ☐ Sea salt
- ☐ Smoked paprika
- ☐ Thyme
- ☐ Turmeric
- ☐ Vanilla extract *(no alcohol added)*

Sweeteners:

- ☐ Grade B maple syrup
- ☐ Raw, unfiltered honey
- ☐ Liquid stevia *(if using)*
- ☐ 1 bag coconut sugar, *(8 ounces)*

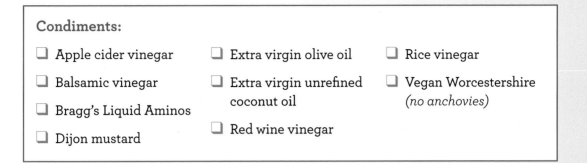

Condiments:

- ❑ Apple cider vinegar
- ❑ Balsamic vinegar
- ❑ Bragg's Liquid Aminos
- ❑ Dijon mustard
- ❑ Extra virgin olive oil
- ❑ Extra virgin unrefined coconut oil
- ❑ Red wine vinegar
- ❑ Rice vinegar
- ❑ Vegan Worcestershire *(no anchovies)*

Other:

- ❑ 2 cartons almond milk
- ❑ 1 jar capers
- ❑ 1 15-ounce can coconut milk
- ❑ 1 jar pitted kalamata olives
- ❑ 1 jar green olives
- ❑ 1 jar roasted red bell peppers
- ❑ 3 packages *(8 ounces each)* tempeh
- ❑ 1 can tomato paste
- ❑ Vegan protein powder of choice *(see Resources section)*
- ❑ 2 boxes low-sodium vegetable broth

Tea and Coffee Substitutes:

- ❑ Dandy Blend *(can buy online)*
- ❑ Herbal teas
- ❑ Roasted dandelion root tea
- ❑ Teeccino *(optional)*

Shopping List: Days 5 to 8

Before shopping for Days 5 to 8, first check what you have on hand before buying everything on this list. I cannot stress this enough. You do not want to over shop and let food spoil. Also, compare what you have on hand to the meal plans for days 4 through 8 as well. You will already have most of the oils/condiments and sweeteners that are needed from your first shop, so you won't need to buy them again. They should last you throughout the 14 days and beyond.

I am only providing you with a shopping list for the first week of the program. The reason I do this is because I want you to learn how to incorporate this way of eating into your lifestyle, so you'll be able to shop on your own once the program is over. Also, you will have some leftover food, and you may want to repeat some meals from the first week because they are so delish! Feel free to do that. It's up to you!

But, again, be sure to schedule in time to make your lists, shop, and prepare yourself for the final week. This is where you will get to see where you may let life get in the way. Remember, one of the biggest SAPs that people have is not planning. This is what can totally throw them, of course. You are now getting the chance to put what you have learned in the first week of the program into action! *I believe in you!* You can do this!

Veggies:

- ❑ 1 bunch asparagus
- ❑ ½ head broccoli
- ❑ 1 bunch carrots
- ❑ 1 cucumber
- ❑ 1 head curly kale
- ❑ 1 small daikon radish
- ❑ 1 bulb garlic
- ❑ 2 large garnet yams
- ❑ 2-inch piece ginger
- ❑ 1 cup green beans
- ❑ 2 red onions
- ❑ 1 yellow onion
- ❑ 2 small red potatoes
- ❑ 3 red bell peppers
- ❑ ½ head red cabbage
- ❑ 1 head romaine lettuce
- ❑ 1 bunch scallions
- ❑ 8 shiitake mushrooms
- ❑ Small spaghetti squash
- ❑ 1 bunch or 7-ounce bag spinach
- ❑ ½ head white cabbage
- ❑ 6 white mushrooms
- ❑ 1 zucchini

Fruits:

- ☐ 1 green apple
- ☐ 1 avocado
- ☐ 2 bananas
- ☐ Fruit of choice for Power Protein Breakfast Bowl and Fruit with Crème Sauce *(see recipe section)*
- ☐ 6 limes
- ☐ 1 12-ounce bag frozen mango

Fresh Herbs:

- ☐ Cilantro
- ☐ Dill
- ☐ Parsley

Spices/Dried Herbs:

- ☐ Basil
- ☐ Cayenne
- ☐ Curry powder
- ☐ Garam masala *(Indian spice)*

Grains/Beans:

- ☐ Gluten-free bread crumbs
- ☐ Brown rice *(if needed)*
- ☐ 2 cans *(15 ounces)* black beans
- ☐ 1 cup dry Puy *(French)* lentils
- ☐ 1 cup dry red lentils

Nuts/Seeds:

- ☐ 1 cup shelled pistachios

Condiments:

- ☐ Sesame oil

Other:

- ☐ 1 jar artichoke hearts
- ☐ 1 can *(12.3 ounces)* coconut milk
- ☐ 1 large carton coconut water
- ☐ 1 8 ounce bag maca *(see Resource Section)*
- ☐ 1 can *(28 ounces)* fire-roasted crushed tomatoes
- ☐ 1 can *(15 ounces)* fire-roasted diced tomatoes
- ☐ 1 bag or jar sundried tomatoes
- ☐ 1 carton low-sodium vegetable broth
- ☐ 1 bag wakame seaweed *(in international aisle)*
- ☐ 1 tub mellow white miso paste *(in refrigerator section)*

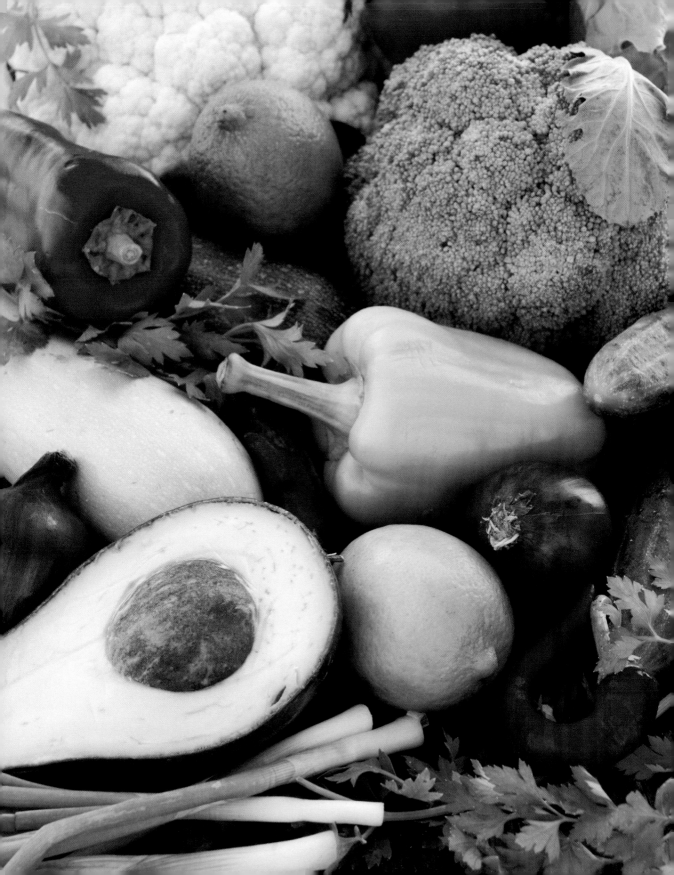

Chapter

8

Clean in 14 Rituals

Each day of the program you will be given a specific focus. This will tie in to the cleanse and support you on your journey. Every morning, read the daily entry and complete the exercises for the day as prompted. Remember to schedule in the time to do this, as I've mentioned earlier in the book. This will ensure that you get the full benefit from this cleanse, and really dig in to any behaviors that may have stopped you in the past from fully stepping into your vital, healthy self. These exercises will also help set you up for the day, and for the entire program.

Isn't it awesome that you will never have to diet again or think about calories? It's so liberating, in my opinion. You will break years of bad habits and get yourself into a place of balance. You will be able to use discernment when making choices for yourself because now you will be informed. How cool is that?

Remember, it will not serve you to skip any steps of this cleanse. I know you want to receive the most benefit, so I say *go for it*—all the way! Put yourself in the game 110 percent! On the last page after Day 14, there is also a round of bonus questions you can answer each day that will consistently be the same. I encourage you to do this, as it will give you good insight into how well you are doing on the cleanse and where you may get off track.

Clean in 14: Week 1

Day 1 Courage

Courage is being scared to death, but saddling up anyway.

—John Wayne

Today is *the* day! You have done all the prep work and now you are at Day 1! You know what that means? *You rock!* I am so proud of you for taking the huge, courageous steps to get here. I know this can feel really scary, and you may not know what to expect. Life is often like that. The unknown can be frightening for many, including me.

There are a lot of tools in this book, so use them. Today's action items will help you kick off your cleanse on the right foot, so to speak. Remember, anything worth doing is never easy. It takes commitment, effort, and courage—and you have all of these! I know this because you picked up this book and are reading this page! Take today step-by-step, minute by minute. If you come up against cravings, sit with them and see what is really there, or make yourself a cup of tea, if the former seems too scary. Your body might be screaming at you, and that's okay. It's part of the process. Stay on track, keep moving forward, and use the tools and exercises provided in this book. Muster up the courage that you have deep inside of you and keep moving forward, no matter what.

Action Items for Day 1

Morning **RITUAL**

Upon Rising: Drink hot lemon water

Morning Kick-Start: 10 cycles of Stress Buster Breaths. Inhale through your nose for a count of 5 and exhale slowly through your mouth for a count of 10. Do this cycle 10 times. This type of breathing engages the parasympathetic nervous system, which helps you to relieve stress and get grounded before your day begins.

An important note: Every time you see the Stress Buster Breaths, follow the same format as given here. You will be given different cycle amounts on different days, but the breathing pattern is the same.

Daily Affirmation: "I am courageous and strong. I can do anything I set my mind to."

Special note: Affirmations are positive statements or confirmations. When repeated, they have a lot of power and can inspire you and literally change your thoughts about yourself. I know this may sound cliché or absurd, but before you judge it, give it a try. Repeating them silently to yourself throughout the day will help you stand stronger in yourself and your commitment to this program and a healthy lifestyle. Even if you don't believe what you are saying 100 percent, they still have power. They only need to be 50 percent believable. This will also shift as you say them more often.

Morning Journal Exercise:

Answer the following five questions (be brutally honest with yourself—this is important):

1 On a scale of 1 to 10 (1 being the lowest and 10 being the highest), how committed am I to my health and well-being?

2 Write three "excuses" or behaviors you are aware of that sabotage your efforts to eat healthy or ways you shortchange yourself.

3 What "reward" do you get (good or bad) when you engage in these behaviors? Examples include: "If I continue to eat unhealthy food, then I will have more time"; "If I continue to eat unhealthy, I will fit in"; or "If I continue to not think about healthy eating, then I don't have to be accountable for my actions." Usually, we will continue with a sabotaging behavior if we are getting some sort of "reward" from it. It keeps us in our unconscious patterns, and Lord knows, the ego does not like to be challenged. Write down your "reward" next to each excuse or behavior.

---

4 What is my intention for this cleanse and beyond (an intention is an expected outcome with positive action attached to it)? Write out your full intention. Here is an example: "My intention is to effortlessly and excitedly enter into this 14-day cleanse with a full commitment to myself while creating delicious, mouthwatering meals and fully utilizing the support available to me. I will take what I learn here and bring it effortlessly into my life moving forward to stay on a healthy, committed path." I know it's long, but it's direct, detailed, and precise. You want to feel it when you write it! Now write yours down and reread it each morning. Take time crafting it. Don't just write anything. Get really clear about what you want your experience to be like during these next few weeks. Just a side note, your intention may change as you go forward in the program. That's okay; just rewrite it and read your new intention each morning.

5 Are there any obstacles in the way of you successfully living out this intention? If so, what are they, and are you willing to let them go?

Evening RITUAL

Evening Journal Exercise:

Flow and Go Writing (10 minutes). Take out your journal and set a timer for 10 minutes. Spend the next 10 minutes writing in your journal in a stream of consciousness, meaning write without filters, judgment, or stopping. Let the pen flow on the paper. Whatever is in your mind, dump it onto the paper. Even if you write, "I don't know what to say, write, whatever. I feel dumb. This is stupid." I mean, *whatever* comes to your mind, dump it on the paper. Drain out everything from your day, all the big and little things, no matter what they are. This is a time to whine, complain, curse, or whatever you need to do to clear your mind. You may even write lists of some sort. There is *no* wrong way to do it. Just *let it flow*. Sometimes I will scribble until more words come. Remember, there is no wrong way. Continue to write for the entire 10 minutes. Once the timer goes off, put down your pen, rip the sheet of paper out of your journal, and shred it or tear it into tiny, tiny pieces and throw it away. Do *not* reread what you have written. Do *not* keep this piece of paper. If something comes to you that is inspirational, copy that specific thought onto another piece of paper for safekeeping.

Relax and Unwind: 10 cycles of Stress Buster Breaths, or a 20-minute guided meditation (To download your free guided meditation, and other bonuses, go to www.karmachow.com/cleanin14bonuses). Good night, sweet one!

Day 2 Pay Attention

Yesterday is history, tomorrow is a mystery, today is a gift.
That's why it's called "the Present."

—Bil Keane

Today may be a rough detox day for you. If you have a headache and feel icky, you are right on track, and it's important that you take really good care of yourself today. If you don't feel any effects from the detox, that's okay too. It doesn't mean anything is wrong or that the cleanse is not working. Remember, our bodies work in different ways, as I have explained earlier in the book, so if you are not having any detox effects, you may get through unscathed, or your body could release later, in layers. No matter how it happens, know that your body is responding how it needs to.

Today's focus is to *pay attention*. Oftentimes we go through our day on autopilot and don't really pay attention to what is happening around us or inside us. We live in the future or past and don't often embrace the present. Today, I want you to really pay attention to your thoughts, feelings, and emotions. I want you to notice what is happening internally, even physically. Paying attention can open you up to new ways of being with yourself. You may start to become aware of feelings you didn't realize were there or sensations that you've never felt before. As you go through the day, check in with yourself and take note of any feelings, sensations, or emotions you have. You will be given an opportunity tonight to write about what you experience.

Action Items for Day 2

Morning **RITUAL**

Upon Rising: Drink hot lemon water

Morning Kick-Start: 10 cycles of Stress Buster Breaths and/or a 10-minute guided meditation

Read Intention

Daily Affirmation: "I am attentive to my own needs and I embrace and accept all that is happening in and around me."

Morning Journal Assignment:

Open your journal and answer the following questions (be specific):

1. What does it mean to you to pay attention?

2. What challenges do you experience during the day that take you out of the present moment or distract you? (This can be reacting to other people, money worries, whatever. Make a list and be as specific as possible.)

3. List three ways you can bring yourself into the present moment and enjoy what is happening to you now (deep breaths, connecting with another person, being thankful for what you do have in your life).

Evening **RITUAL**

Evening Journal Exercise:

Answer the following questions with as much detail as possible:

1. How did I feel today (physically, emotionally, and mentally)? What did I notice about paying attention? Was it easy? Challenging? Be specific.

> **2** Did anything in particular stick out for me today that felt different than every other day? If so, what was it?

Relax and Unwind: 10 cycles of Stress Buster Breaths and/or a 20-minute guided meditation. Sweet dreams!

Day 3   Strength

You can always take the easy way out and give up,
but real strength comes when you decide to keep pushing
forward no matter what the circumstances are.

—Unknown

You've made it to Day 3. That's a huge accomplishment! The first part of this program will be the hardest, and once you get further into it, it will begin to fly by, especially as you feel your body, energy, and moods begin to shift.

Today's focus is *strength.* And I don't mean physical strength. I am referring to a strength that is deep inside of you, similar to the courage I talked about on Day 1. This strength is something we all have, and we usually rely on it or utilize it when we are going through unexpected hard times.

As you go through your day, I want you to tap into that inner strength that resides in you. It's the part of you that says "no" when you have a craving for sugar. Or the part of you that musters up the energy to work out, even when you don't feel like it, or to continue on, even when you want to quit. It's *in you.* Even though it's not tangible, it's there. Each time you feel a twinge today of wanting to give up or give in because this feels scary or hard, dig deep down into that inner strength and remember your Big Why and reason for doing this program. Even if you flub up and eat something you are not supposed to, or give in to a craving, go to your inner strength to hop back on the horse and continue forward versus letting your SAPs get the better of you.

Action Items for Day 3

Morning **RITUAL**

Upon Rising: Drink hot lemon water

Morning Kick-Start: 10 cycles of Stress Buster Breaths and/or 10-minute guided meditation

Read Intention

Daily Affirmation: "I am strong and willing to make positive, permanent change. I have power over my own life."

Morning Journal Assignment: Zap the SAP

1 List your top three most sabotaging addictive patterns when it comes to your health (e.g., not planning, eating sweets, eating on the go, etc.).

2 Beside each behavior, write down ways or ideas you have about how you can change them.

3 Today, take one contrary action (doing the opposite of what you would normally do) against a sabotaging behavior (e.g., if you normally reach for sweets after lunch, make yourself a cup of tea, or do some Morning Kick-Start instead). Write about this in your evening journal assignment.

Evening **RITUAL**

Evening Journal Assignment: Part 1

1 Write about the contrary action you took today when it came to your sabotaging behavior. What was it? How did it feel to take this action? What did you notice in your body and in the way you felt, emotionally and mentally? Be specific.

---

② Write one word describing how your life would feel without this specific behavior (write it in capital letters and circle it). Repeat this word silently to yourself 10 times. Breathe it in and feel it in your body. This will help to begin the rewiring process of this sabotaging behavior.

Evening Journal Assignment: Part 2

Answer the following questions in your journal. Be specific when answering:

① How well did I follow the plan today?

② How did I feel about what I was eating? Did I feel satisfied? Deprived? Hungry?

③ Did I feel self-conscious about being on the cleanse when around others? If so, why? What thoughts or emotions came up for me regarding food today? How did I handle them?

④ Did I do the best I could today with regards to this program? If not, what could I do differently tomorrow to be sure I am on track?

Relax and Unwind: 10 cycles of Stress Buster Breaths and/or a 20-minute guided meditation. Nighty night!

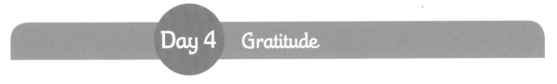

Day 4   Gratitude

If the only prayer you ever said was thank you,
that would be enough.

—Meister Eckhart

Yesterday you focused a little bit on shifting sabotaging behaviors. Today we are going to focus on the positive things in our life through practicing *gratitude*. Too often we can get wrapped up in the negative things that are happening around us or to us, and this can send us in a downward spiral. I know that when I start to talk negatively to myself, it takes me into a deep, dark hole that seems impossible to climb out of. The quickest way I shift this is by focusing on all the things in my life, or on that specific day, that I have to be thankful for.

Gratitude is one of the quickest ways to bring us present, along with conscious breathing. When you put your attention on something that is positive, you cannot be in the negative. Love and hate cannot exist at the same time. Anger and joy cannot exist at the same time. So when you put your mind toward the things you are grateful for, it's hard to be in a negative state, and you will naturally feel more joyful and happy.

Action Items for Day 4

Morning RITUAL

Upon Rising: Drink hot lemon water

Morning Kick-Start: 10 cycles of Stress Buster Breaths and/or a 10-minute guided meditation

Read Intention

Daily Affirmation: "I am truly grateful for all the beautiful blessings in my life. Thank you. Thank you. Thank you."

Morning Journal Assignment

Make a numbered list from 1 to 5 in your journal. Write down five things in your life that you are grateful for. They don't have to be elaborate. It can be as simple as "I am grateful for my bed." Once you are done, go back and read each of them three times. As you read them, see if you can feel the gratitude in your heart. Think of that person, place, or thing with loving-kindness, and smile as you do this. I guarantee your whole state will shift. What an awesome way to start your day!

Bonus Activity: As you go through your day today, do your best to notice and be aware of all the blessings around you. See if you can be in an attitude of gratitude today for all of these things.

Evening Journal Assignment:

1 Did you notice any change in the way you felt today versus yesterday? If so, what was it?

2 Did you participate in the bonus activity? If so, were you able to actually feel gratitude? How did it feel? Did you notice if your mood shifted?

3 What does gratitude mean to you? Be specific.

4 Does saying your affirmation throughout the day feel supportive? Why or why not?

Relax and Unwind: 10 cycles of Stress Buster Breaths and/or a 20-minute guided meditation. Sleep well, sweet friend!

Day 5   Living on Purpose

Your purpose in life is to find your purpose and
give your whole heart and soul to it.

—Buddha

As you go through this program, you may experience a lot of change, not only physically but also emotionally and mentally. I created this program to be well rounded because I believe vital health doesn't just stem from what we eat and if we get exercise or not. It stems from many things, such as managing our stress, our thoughts, the way we feel, and so on. There are too many people in the world who live their lives for others and not themselves. They work at a dead-end job, or they feel trapped in other areas of their life without any escape. Some people are trapped by their eating habits or obsessive thoughts about their bodies. Whatever it is, we can create a self-imposed prison if we are not careful to live our lives on purpose.

Living on purpose means that you are actually making choices about your life and not letting life take charge. You are at the helm, steering the ship that is your life. You can keep it on course or let it veer off, but *you* are the captain. You get to make the decisions each day regarding your own health and well-being. And remember—there are consequences to every decision you make, whether "good" or "bad." So it's best to make an informed decision out of discernment.

Action Items for Day 5

Morning RITUAL

Upon Rising: Drink hot lemon water

Morning Kick-Start: 10 cycles of Stress Buster Breaths and/or a 10-minute guided meditation

Read Intention

Daily Affirmation: "I am in charge of my life. I am captain of my body and health. I make decisions that are purposeful and serve my highest good."

Morning Journal Assignment: None

Evening RITUAL

Move It: Set a timer for 15 minutes. Roll out a yoga mat or workout mat. Stretch and move your body however it feels it needs it. This could be forward bends, twists, feet up the wall. Play around. Breathe into the places that feel stiff or stuck. Pain is simply stuck energy in the body that has built up over time and needs to move. Stretching, along with using your breath, will gently help to move this energy.

In a short paragraph, describe what "living life on purpose" means to you. Once you have done this, ask yourself if you are, in fact, living your life on purpose. If the answer is "no," write down three small steps you can take toward living more purposefully. For example, if you are passionate about horses but have never worked with them, a small step toward accomplishing your dream would be to do some research online about how you could interact with horses in your area. Every small step you take toward a more purposeful life makes a difference. If you feel like you are already living your life on purpose in every way, then kudos to you! You are on track! Sleep peacefully, sweet friend.

Day 6 Go Gently

Oh! That gentleness! How far more potent is it than force!
—Charlotte Brontë, *Jane Eyre*

It's Day 6 and I am *so* proud of how far you have come. You have almost completed a week, which means that you are almost halfway through the program! Doesn't that feel amazing?

Today, I want you to focus on *being gentle* with yourself. You have been doing so amazingly well over these last few days, so it's time to take care of yourself, gently. You may not know what this means, as being gentle can feel foreign to many of us. Oftentimes our inner dialogue is less than gentle, and we can say things to ourselves that are not supportive or nice. This is how we sabotage ourselves and our efforts. If we do one little thing that we perceive as less than perfect, we oftentimes berate ourselves or just give up. Remember what I said about perfection in the first part of the book? It sucks!

I know when I am not feeling up to par, my negative self-talk kicks in, and I feel as though nothing can get me out of it. It's these times when I have learned to be very gentle with myself and not judge myself as bad for feeling this way. It's part of life sometimes. I find what helps is doing something that fills my soul, like heading to the beach, going for a walk, or playing with my dog. These actions shift my state and bring me to a gentler place inside.

Action Items for Day 6

Morning **RITUAL**

Upon Rising: Drink hot lemon water

Morning Kick-Start: 10 cycles of Stress Buster Breaths and/or a 10-minute guided meditation

Read Intention

Daily Affirmation: "I am worthy of slowing down and putting my needs before others' needs."

Morning Journal Assignment:

Zap the *SAPs*. In your journal make a list of all the negative things you say to yourself throughout the day. You may be thinking, *I don't do that*. Yet often, subconsciously, we have a script running that doesn't always contain the nicest thoughts about ourselves. For example, if you mess something up, do you call yourself stupid or a failure? Take a few moments and think about what your regular negative self-talk is. For me, when I get dressed in the morning, I oftentimes say, "Oh god, I hate my thighs." This is a perfect example of the negative self-talk that is ingrained in me, and that I need to practice shifting. The more I hate my thighs, the uglier and uglier they will get. I know this may sound odd, but our bodies do actually respond to us by following our lead, whether negative or positive.

Once you are done with the list, I want you to reframe each item on the list by writing a positive spin on the put-down. For example, I would write, "I am grateful for my thighs and legs because they are strong and carry me throughout my day, on hikes and long walks with my dog."

Once you are done reframing each item, go back and read them over two times, then put your journal away. Make a promise to yourself, over the next 24 hours, to catch yourself each time you participate in negative self-talk, and say to yourself, "That's not even remotely true." This practice will start to switch your negative thinking about yourself.

> ### Evening Journal Assignment
>
> Make a list in your journal of things you can do to shift your state when you get into a negative mind-set. I listed mine in the introductory paragraph, so what are yours? Once you list them, pick the top three that you could see yourself doing and circle them. I want you to write these three down on a small Post-it note and put it in your wallet to carry around with you. When you get into a negative mind-set or start talking bad to yourself, pull out your top three and take an action listed there. Do this as often as you need to!

Relax and Unwind: 10 cycles of Stress Buster Breaths or a 20-minute nighttime meditation. Sweetest of dreams, cleanse warrior!

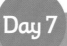

Day 7   Ask for What You Need

*Each time we face our fears, we gain strength,
courage, and confidence in the doing.*

—Anonymous

It's the last day of Week 1! I am hopeful that you are over the detox hump by now and starting to really feel the positive changes of this program. You might be feeling more energetic, even-keeled, focused, and lighter.

Your focus today is to practice *asking for what you need*. Sadly, this doesn't always come naturally, especially for women. We have been conditioned to do everything on our own, and asking for help can feel like we are weak or incapable. This has been a huge lesson for me in my lifetime and not something that has come easy to me.

I have learned over the years to ask for help, or ask for what I need. And I have to say, learning this has changed my life tremendously in that it's made my life easier, more manageable in times of stress, and has helped me feel more connected. I have discovered through this that others do like to help us, and if they don't, we have to trust them enough to say no. If they can't say no, and they do it out of guilt or to please us, then that's on them.

I can't tell you how many times I've moved over the last 20 years, only to find myself doing it all alone and feeling frustrated, angry, and resentful that none of my friends would help me. But guess what? I never asked them to. I just assumed they would offer to help because I had mentioned it one time in passing.

So today, focus on asking for what you need. I know this can be challenging and may make you feel vulnerable. You may find yourself being afraid of someone saying no, or the possibility of feeling rejected. The way I see it is if someone says no, they are giving us a gift. They are honoring themselves, and we don't have to take it personally. On to the next, right? And it also teaches us to not be attached to a specific outcome, which can also be challenging.

I practice this a lot at restaurants, especially because I do eat a "special" diet (funny that healthy is considered "special." Hopefully one day it will be the norm). I have found that more often than not, when I ask from my heart, and not from a place of self-righteousness, I always receive what I need and more so. People are willing and want to help! So today *ask for what you need*. Come on. Just do it and see what happens.

Action Items for Day 7

Morning RITUAL

Upon Rising: Drink hot lemon water

Morning Kick-Start: 10 cycles of Stress Buster Breaths or a 10-minute guided meditation

Read Intention

Daily Affirmation: "I deserve to ask for what I need/want. It shows my strength and vulnerability."

Morning Journal Assignment:

In your journal, answer the following questions:

1. If I ask for what I need, and someone says no, what meaning do I give that?
2. If I ask for help, does that mean I am weak or incapable?
3. Do I often do things myself because it's easier than asking for help or because I can get it done more quickly on my own?

If you answered yes to any of these, this is a good time to reflect on where you might be trying to control many areas of your life. Are you willing to give up control to let others help you, even if they don't do it exactly as you would? Make a list of things in your life that you need help with or would like support with but have been too afraid to reach out or ask for. Read the list over, pick one that feels really big, and ask someone today to help you with it. Even if it's just saying, "I am thinking about doing this thing, and I would love your support." See how you feel after.

Evening **RITUAL**

Evening Journal Assignment:

In your journal, write about your experience with asking for help/support or what you need. Be detailed and specific. Will you do it again? How did you feel when doing it? What emotions rose up in you while you were asking?

Relax and Unwind: 10 cycles of Stress Buster Breaths and/or a 20-minute guided meditation.

Week 1 Wrap-Up

I know that you really dove in this week and gave it your all. I'm guessing it was probably very overwhelming for you at first. Remember what I said in the beginning of the book, that if you are scared, it means something to you? Changing a routine or a way of living can be hard. Your ego *hates* change, and it will do anything to keep you living exactly the way you have been, even if it's not healthy for you. In fact, the ego thrives on drama and ill ways of being.

So I want you to take a few minutes to acknowledge yourself and all the huge steps you have made this week. I want you to relish in how far you've come and the changes that you have instilled in yourself so far. How do you feel? Do you feel like you have accomplished something big? Well, you better, because *you have*. Now, on to Week 2. You're coming down the homestretch! You're so cool!

Clean in 14: Week 2

It's Week 2 and you are halfway through the program! I am doing a happy dance for you! Seriously, you have made it through the hardest part, and now it's about digging down deep and continuing the forward movement that you have gained. You've got this—I have *no* doubt! You are a true, courageous warrior and someone who takes themselves seriously, and I commend you.

Hopefully this week will flow much easier for you, as you are more in the groove now. You will still be engaging in daily assignments, so don't skip over them, because they are really important to your journey during this program. By doing them each day, you will be shifting patterns so you can move forward after the program without any hesitancy and bad habits lingering. You will finish off with strength and an inner knowledge that you may not have had before. You may even want to revisit your original intention and see if it has changed at all. If it has, rewrite it and keep it in your journal for your daily morning rituals.

Day 8   Trust Yourself

*We all have a better guide in ourselves, if we would attend to it,
than any other person can be.*

—Jane Austen, *Mansfield Park*

Today's focus is a big one and one that you may be unfamiliar with. We often move through life listening to what others say and doing things that others want us to do, especially our parents or family members. Sometimes the requests asked of us don't make us feel good inside, yet we do them anyway, only to kick ourselves or be resentful later. We have a hard time saying no because we feel bad or that we "should" participate even if we don't necessarily want to.

This is what I mean about trusting yourself. Each of us has a still, small voice within that always knows the next right step, and if we slow down enough to listen and take action from that place, we are usually in alignment. If we are taking action from the place of our ego, or from a place inside that doesn't feel good, then we do not trust ourselves.

Sometimes it can be hard to discern between what is ego and what is intuition or inner knowing. Usually we can feel something intuitively in our gut or our heart. It's usually a signal from our body that is telling us what to do or what decision to make. The problem is that so many of us are out of touch with our bodies that we cannot even feel these intuitive hits. This can happen from years of being hurt, going through challenges, eating bad food, and so on. It's all connected. It takes practice to tune in to what our bodies are really trying to tell us. Today's exercises are about getting you back in touch with your intuition, trusting yourself, and looking at some SAPs that are keeping you from following your gut.

Action Items for Day 8

Morning **RITUAL**

Upon Rising: Drink hot lemon water

Morning Kick-Start: 10 cycles of Stress Buster Breaths and/or a 10-minute guided meditation

Read Intention

Daily Affirmation: "I listen to that small, still voice within and trust that I have all the answers I need inside."

Morning Journal Assignment:

In your journal, write a list of things you have done in the last few months that you really didn't want to do but did anyway. Next to each item, write how you felt before, during, and after. Now write what you would've preferred to do instead, for example, get a pedicure instead of taking your friend to the airport, or watch a sports game instead of helping your friend move. You get the idea.

Evening **RITUAL**

Evening Journal Assignment

Zap the *SAP*. Oftentimes we have subconscious patterns running inside of us that we are not completely aware of. These patterns keep us stuck and may keep us from fully trusting our own intuition, or even hearing our intuition. Open your journal and write down two or three patterns that you are aware of, or have a sense of, that keep you stuck or that keep coming up for you in your life. For me, whenever I am sad or feel emotional, I turn to food and sabotage all my healthy eating efforts. Or, to take it a step deeper, sometimes when life is going too well, I will do something (unconsciously, of course) that will feel bad. These ways of being can sometimes be so ingrained in us that we don't even know they are happening. Yet most of us have some sort of awareness regarding our patterns, and hopefully this program has brought you more in touch with yours.

After writing these patterns down, next to each one write the ways in which you can see how they cause you to not trust yourself, or even to trust others. See if you can tune in to where each of these patterns stemmed from, or track back to the first time you actually felt a certain way and engaged in the pattern. For example, your mom yelled at you and you turned to food. I know that this can be a bit scary to go into, and if you are not ready to do it, that's okay. You can always come back to it when you feel ready. Writing about these patterns actually helps to shift them and get more in touch with ourselves. See if you can get a sense of that. You don't have to do anything further, just notice what is happening. You can also reach out on the Clean in 14 Facebook board if you need more support.

Relax and Unwind: 10 cycles of of Stress Buster Breaths and/or a 20-minute guided meditation. Sleep peacefully.

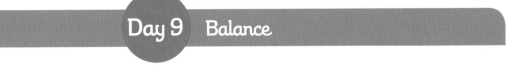

Day 9   Balance

Life is a balanced system of learning and evolution.
Whether pleasure or pain, every situation in your life serves a purpose.
It is up to us to recognize what that purpose could be.
—Steve Maraboli

Ah, *balance*. It's something most of us strive for but rarely ever experience. I have come to realize that it's super easy to let life get out of balance and super hard to keep it in balance. I wonder why that is? Well, oftentimes we have certain things in our life that require more of our attention than others. Whether it is a job, children, or whatever, we tend to focus our attention on one or two specific areas of our lives more than others, and that can create imbalance. What usually happens for me when I let my life get extremely out of balance is that I pay for it with ill health. This is usually the case for most, because healthy eating and exercise are usually the first things we let go of in lieu of everything else.

Taking care of ourselves is a constant practice, and requires dedication and commitment. After you are done with this program, I wouldn't expect you to just give up on yourself and go back to your old ways. Even though you actually might, you will have many more tools after completing this program than you had before, so making that decision will be one of discernment on your part. There are ways to have balance in our lives; it's just a matter of figuring out what's really important to us. I am not saying that we will have total balance all the time, but if we can get our lives to a place where we feel happy and in the flow, that's a really good thing. To get to this place, we need to put rituals into place, which is what I meant by maintaining a daily practice. Whether it's exercise, meditation, time alone, doing things we love, or other actions, we must engage in these activities on a regular basis to keep our center. When we are centered and grounded in ourselves, it doesn't matter if life gets out of balance, because we are balanced within. I know that when I have a sense of being centered, I handle life much more gracefully, and the nonsensical stuff tends to fall away. I am easier to be around, I have more energy, and I feel more motivated to focus on the things that matter. So this might help you understand how important it is to take care of yourself and do things that nurture you. Remember, it doesn't happen overnight, but each small step you take every day leads to a big change down the road.

Action Items for Day 9

Morning RITUAL

Upon Rising: Drink hot lemon water

Morning Kick-Start: 10 cycles of Stress Buster Breaths and/or a 10-minute guided meditation

Read Intention

Daily Affirmation: "I make self-honoring choices that will provide balance in all areas of my life."

Morning Journal Assignment:

In your journal write out the following words:

- Career
- Finances
- Personal growth/spirituality
- Family
- Health
- Relationships/friends
- Social life/fun
- Attitude

Now, next to each topic, rate them from 1 to 10 (1 being the lowest and 10 being the highest), as to where they stand in your life in terms of satisfaction. Be honest here—this is important. If you don't put energy into your health and you feel lousy all the time, you might rate it between 1 and 3. You get the idea. Now take a look at the numbers. Any topic with a number below 5 needs your attention and is considered out of balance with the other areas of your life.

Next, write each topic that is under 5 in a separate section and leave some space. Under each topic, write three action steps you can take to start to bring that part of your life closer to a 10. Over the next two weeks, focus on putting these steps into action. You can either write them on your calendar or your to-do list, but whatever you do, make them happen. Maybe you could even practice Day 7's focus and ask for some support from your friends and family.

Evening RITUAL

Evening Journal Assignment:

Open your journal and reread your entry from this morning. See if anything else stands out to you. If so, write more action steps or change some things. Once you are done, get out your schedule and set aside a minimum of 15 minutes three times in the coming week to focus on any action steps you wrote down for your "under 5" topics.

Relax and Unwind: 10 cycles of Stress Buster Breaths and/or a 20-minute guided meditation.

Day 10 Slow Down and Tune In

Slow down and everything you are chasing
will come around and catch you.

—John De Paola

Slowing down is not something Americans do very well. With all the technology today, we are constantly bombarded with news, ads, information, you name it. Cell phones and e-mail keep us accessible 24/7, which never really allows us time to disconnect or slow down. We eat in the car, on the run, or standing over the kitchen sink—guilty! Life has become unmanageable for many.

I have been working with a private client for the last couple months who is a mother of two, has a full-time job, and is completely overwhelmed. She has given over to the fact that her life is never going to slow down. Though she has a husband and her mother-in-law lives right down the street, she feels she can't ask for help and that she needs to do everything herself. This is a trap we get caught in. If we live with this attitude, we will become a victim of our circumstances. This is also the curse of perfectionism or another way we try to control every facet of our life.

It's important that we make a conscious effort to slow down, unplug, and spend quality time with ourselves. This may often include asking others for help or being willing to reprioritize and let go of some things in your life that may not be serving you, like spending two hours on Facebook a day or watching eight hours of TV per week.

Being overloaded can disconnect us, not only from others but from ourselves as well. We become numb and out of touch with our bodies and the way we feel. We are constantly looking to the next thing to occupy us and numb us—whether it's Facebook, games on your phone, watching TV, overeating or drinking alcohol, you name it. We all find ways to numb ourselves, and in turn, we get out of tune with ourselves, and our bodies.

Today is all about *slowing down and tuning in* to how you feel and what your body, mind, and soul need. This might be hard for you. It takes practice. Tuning in daily for short periods of time will start to bring you in touch with your body so that you can hear what it needs versus what your ego/mind thinks it wants. So take the time today to really tune in to yourself and notice what your body is telling you.

Action Items for Day 10

Morning RITUAL

Upon Rising: Drink hot lemon water

Morning Kick-Start: 15 cycles of Stress Buster Breaths and/or a 10-minute guided meditation

Read Intention

Daily Affirmation: "I am more valuable to myself and to others when I slow down, tune in, and take time to smell the roses."

Morning Journal Assignment:

Make a list of ways you might check out and/or distract yourself (e.g., hours on Facebook, watching TV, drinking alcohol, constantly checking e-mail, etc.). This is not meant to make you feel bad; it's about taking an honest look at your life and where you may be expending time that you could otherwise use more sensibly.

Evening RITUAL

Evening Journal Assignment:

Set a timer for 15 minutes. Write down what it means to you to slow down (be as specific and detailed as possible). Sometimes people stay busy because it helps them to feel of value. Does this seem like you? Do you have fear that if you slow down you will become lazy or feel too much? We can often distract ourselves and stay busy because we are running from our feelings and ourselves. How did you feel today when you were slowing down and tuning in? What did you notice? Write about this until your timer runs out.

Relax and Unwind: 10 cycles of Stress Buster Breaths and/or a 20-minute guided meditation. Nighty night!

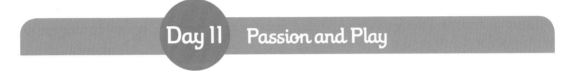

Day 11 Passion and Play

Play is the only way the highest intelligence of humankind can unfold.
—Joseph Chilton Pearce

It's Day 11, and we are coming down the homestretch. I hope you are feeling a spring in your step. You may also be getting compliments from coworkers, family members, and friends who want to know why you are so energetic and your eyes are so bright! You only have three days left, but remember—you can feel this way for a lifetime. It doesn't end here.

Today's focus is on *passion* and *play*. So, I want to know, what are you *passionate* about? What do you like to do for fun? What makes you laugh? Passion and play are such an important part of living a healthy, happy life. If you don't make time for the things that bring you joy and laughter, and that you feel a deep passion for, life may feel empty, long, and challenging. Having passion keeps us healthy.

Have you let your passion for life fall away? Have you gotten stuck in a rut and stopped doing the things that you love or that feel good to you? Do you even remember what it was that you felt passionate about? Do you give everyone else your time—except yourself? If you are nodding your head right now, then maybe it's time to get busy playing!

As adults we can become a bit too serious and don't leave any time for playing or engaging in activities for which we feel passion. Today's assignments will help you tap into that place of play and passion. So let's have some fun!

Action Items for Day 11

Morning **RITUAL**

Upon Rising: Drink hot lemon water

Morning Kick-Start: 15 cycles of Stress Buster Breaths and/or a 10-minute guided meditation

Read Intention

Daily Affirmation: "I give myself permission to play, laugh, and feel passionate about life."

Morning Journal Assignment:

Make a list of things you loved to do as a child. Make a list of things you love to do as an adult but don't make time for. Reread both lists and circle those activities/things that resonate most with you, that you feel you have a longing or yearning for.

Evening **RITUAL**

Evening Journal Assignment:

Take one action step toward one of the circled items on your list. Whether it's scheduling in a basketball game with your buddies, going to the art store, or doing research online, take the action tonight to get the ball rolling!

Relax and Unwind: 10 cycles of Stress Buster Breaths and/or a 20-minute guided meditation. Sleep playfully.

Day 12　Self-Appreciation

Nothing builds self-esteem and self-confidence like accomplishment.

—Thomas Carlyle

It's Day 12! Only two more days to go! Wow, I am so inspired by you and blown away by your commitment to your health and well-being! Self-appreciation is something that most people may think of as conceited or arrogant, but I find it to be just the opposite. It's humbling, and a way for us to show up for ourselves so that we can show up better for others.

Today is all about *appreciating yourself*, to acknowledge yourself for how far you have come in this program and in life. Self-appreciation is as important as passion for keeping us healthy and happy. You may never tell yourself how proud you are of yourself, so I am going to do it now: *I am proud of you!*

By acknowledging ourselves, we show up in the world happier and healthier. It's not boastful; it's loving and self-nurturing. We can be of better service to others when we take care of and appreciate ourselves first.

Action Items for Day 12

Morning **RITUAL**

Upon Rising: Drink hot lemon water

Morning Kick-Start: 15 cycles of Stress Buster Breaths and/or a 10-minute guided meditation

Read Intention

Daily Affirmation: "I love, accept and appreciate myself exactly as I am in this moment. I am perfect in all my imperfection."

Morning Journal Assignment:

Open your journal to a blank page and number the page from 1 to 10. Put a smile on your face. Now, write down ten things you value/appreciate about yourself (be specific and go deep,) using the "I am" format. For example, "I am an awesome listener." Once you are done with your list, reread it three times, *slowly*, while breathing deeply, and then put it away. Notice what you feel when doing this. Once you are done, write a short paragraph about what you noticed when reading these awesome things about yourself. Did you have judgment? Did you feel silly? Did you feel boastful or egotistical? Write down what came up.

Now pick your top three and write them down on a separate sheet in your journal. Rip it out and hang it in a place where you can see it every day. Repeat these self-appreciation mantras silently to yourself throughout the day and see how your attitude begins to shift.

Evening RITUAL

Evening Journal Assignment:

Take out your list from this morning. Reread it again. How do you feel now when you read the list? Does your list still resonate from this morning? If not, take the time now to change it. Do all the items on your list reflect things you do for other people and not really things you like about yourself? Oftentimes, the things we appreciate about ourselves are focused outside of us, like giving to others, always showing up for others, being a good friend to others, and so on. See if you can turn inward and choose things that are self-focused, like "I am a good friend to myself," or "I am strong," or "I am an awesome communicator." There is no right or wrong here. I just want you to notice and dig in to this exercise to see if you can take it to a deeper level and get to the things that you really do believe and appreciate about yourself, not what others appreciate about you. Take about 15 minutes to complete this assignment and reflect. Write about whatever comes up for you.

Relax and Unwind: 10 cycles of Stress Buster Breaths and/or a 20-minute guided meditation.

Day 13   Connection

We cannot live only for ourselves. A thousand fibers connect us with our fellow men; and among those fibers, as sympathetic threads, our actions run as causes, and they come back to us as effects.

—Herman Melville

Connection is something that human beings crave but often shy away from. We need connection to thrive in all areas of our life. In the technology age, even though we feel more connected through certain social media venues, studies are showing that we are even more disconnected from ourselves and others because we've confused communication with connection. We have less face time with people, and we often spend more time with our heads buried in our cell phones, laptops, and so on. To me, this is a pandemic, especially among school-age kids and teens. Soon enough, humans will not know how to interact with one another at all, and won't be receiving the nurturing and emotional support we need for growth and brain development.

Spending time with other human beings and having intimate connections is extremely important for our health and spiritual growth. Many of us feel like we have to do everything on our own, or that we are truly alone in the world, and if we ask for help, we are viewed as weak or incapable.

Today's rituals will be focused on connecting with yourself and others. If this scares you, then I encourage you to move forward with 100 percent commitment. It is through the hardest and scariest times that we grow the most.

Action Items for Day 13

Morning **RITUAL**

Upon Rising: Drink hot lemon water

Morning Kick-Start: 15 cycles of Stress Buster Breaths and/or a 10-minute guided meditation

Read Intention

Daily Affirmation: "I am deeply connected to myself and the world around me. I feel fulfilled when I am connected to others."

Open your journal and write down what it means to you to feel connected, whether to yourself or others. Next, write down ways you keep yourself from being connected to yourself or others in your life. For example, watching hours of TV, playing games on your smartphone, or thinking you may be a burden to others. These are all ways we disconnect. Yes, sometimes we need downtime and time to engage in mindless activity, but we can get carried away and become isolated if we don't make the effort to connect. I love to connect to myself by being out in nature or at the ocean. Exercise is a great way to connect to yourself and your body. So is healthy eating. As you go through your day today, notice any little things you may do that keep you from connecting to others.

Evening **RITUAL**

Evening Journal Assignment:

Take 15 minutes and write about what you noticed today regarding things you did to be disconnected from others. Now write a short list of some actions you can take instead that would result in connection. For example, something I do a lot is e-mail someone instead of picking up the phone, yet I always, always, always feel so much better and more connected when I actually get to talk to a person, or even better, see them.

Relax and Unwind: 10 cycles of Stress Buster Breaths and/or a 20-minute guided meditation. Sleep well, rock star!

Day 14 Celebration

The man who thinks he can and the man who thinks he can't are both right. Which one are you?

—Henry Ford

Today is the last day of the Clean in 14 Program, and it's your day to *celebrate*! Today I want you to really think about how far you've come, how much you've learned, and where you want to go from here.

Celebrating is all about acknowledging our journey and our growth. You have been practicing self-appreciation, so I know it feels like second hat to you by now (wink, wink), so go ahead and celebrate your *huge* accomplishment.

As you go through the day today, think about where you want to go from here and what you want your life to feel like. Just think about it as you relish the last day of the Clean in 14 Program, and how all of your dedication and commitment has paid off.

Action Items for Day 14

Morning **RITUAL**

Upon Rising: Drink hot lemon water

Morning Kick-Start: 15 cycles of Stress Buster Breaths and/or a 10-minute guided meditation

Read Intention

Daily Affirmation: "I celebrate life. I celebrate me. I am awesome and powerful!"

Morning Journal Assignment: None!

Evening **RITUAL**

Impeccable Self-Care Celebratory Action

Do one self-care action tonight before you go to bed that will feel celebratory to you. Whether it's taking a bath, scheduling a massage for later in the week, or listening to your favorite song, do that thing that will feel really good to your soul. *You did it!*

Evening Journal Assignment:

Open your journal. Take a few moments and really think about where you want to go moving forward, how you want your life to look and feel. Do you want to feel healthy, happy, and energetic? Do you want to feel free from food addiction? What are all the things you want internally for yourself and how do you want to feel in your life?

Take about 15 to 20 minutes and write about this. If you have fears that come up, that's okay. It's all part of the process. Write about those fears, too. As you write, see if you can get clearer about how you want life to feel, how you want to live your life, and how you want to show up for people. When you are done writing, read over what you have written and take it all in. Take in the fact that you have completed a 14-day program that you committed yourself to. You really did it!

Relax and Unwind: 10 cycles of Stress Buster Breaths and/or a 20-minute guided meditation.

BONUS • DAILY REFLECTION QUESTIONS

The following bonus questions are here for you to do daily each evening, if you really want to take the program to the next level. Answering them will give you great insight into how you are doing and where you may need to make some changes or shifts.

1 How well did I follow the plan today? How did I feel about what I was eating? Did I feel satisfied? Deprived? Hungry?

2 Did I feel self-conscious about being on the cleanse when around others? If so, why? What thoughts or emotions came up for me around food today? How did I handle them?

3 Did I do the best I could today with regards to this program? If not, what could I do differently tomorrow to be sure I am on track?

Chapter 9

The Recipes

Mostly all of the recipes provided here are simple. I recognize that you may not be someone who spends a lot of time in the kitchen, so my wish is that doing this program opens up a new love of cooking for you.

If you already spend time in the kitchen, then you will most likely feel comfortable with these recipes but you may be introduced to some new foods you have never heard of or thought to use before. Whatever your level in the kitchen, do your best to have fun and make sure you plan your cooking days so that you can be fully present while making these delicious recipes. I love to infuse my food with tons of love as I'm cooking, and although this may sound kind of strange to some people, it really helps me to be more grateful for how much abundance is in front of me.

Breakfast
and Shakes

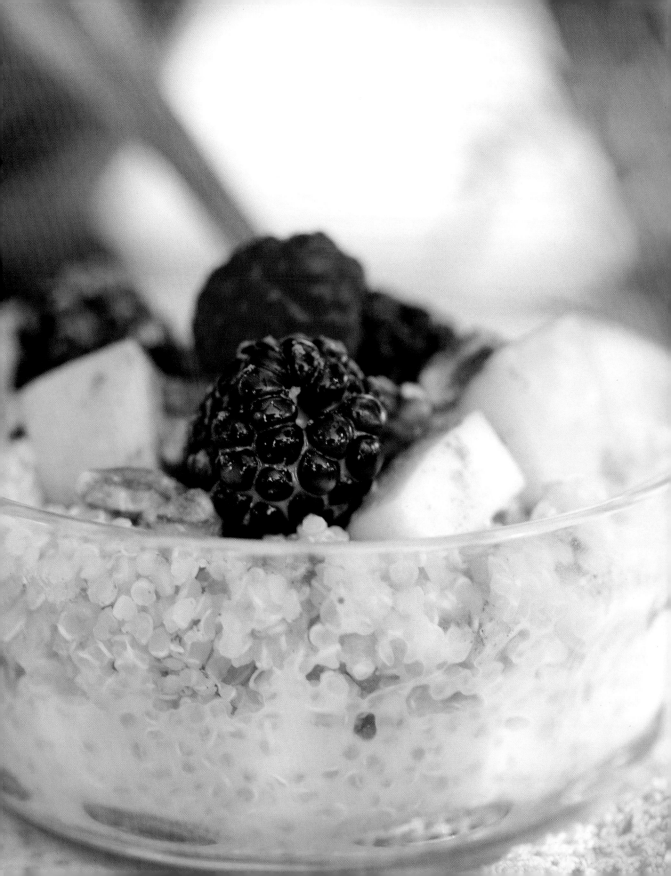

Power Protein Breakfast Bowl

This breakfast bowl is not only filling, it's delicious too.
Quinoa is a perfect protein on its own. It's mostly recognized
as a grain, but it's really a seed. It's considered a superfood in
the Incan culture and is used to maintain energy levels—
a great way to start off your day!

1) In a large bowl, mix together the quinoa,
   apple, hemp seeds, flax seed, oil, pecans,
   cinnamon, and nutmeg. Top with the
   almond milk and a drizzle of syrup
   or honey.

1 Serving

⅔ cup cooked **quinoa**

½ **green apple**, chopped, *or*
   ½ cup **fresh berries**

2 teaspoons **hemp seeds**

2 teaspoons **ground flax seed**

1 teaspoon **coconut oil**, melted

1 handful **raw pecans**

½ teaspoon **cinnamon**

⅛ teaspoon **nutmeg**

Almond milk, unsweetened

Drizzle of **grade B maple syrup**
   or **raw, unfiltered honey**

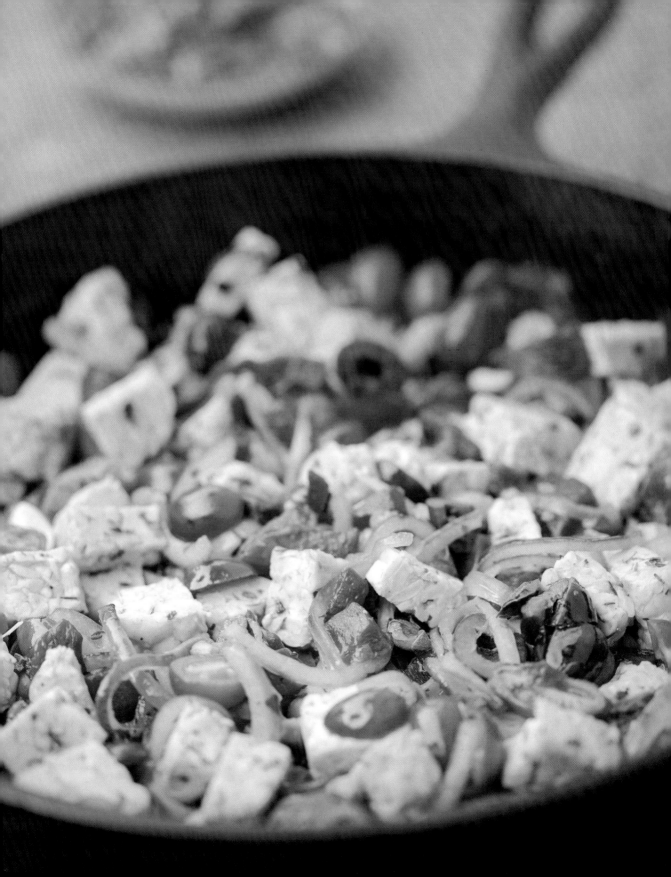

Mediterranean Veggie Scramble

This very flavorful, high-energy veggie scramble is loaded with phytonutrients and protein. It will transport you right to the Greek Isles, it's that good.

1) Heat the oil in a large skillet over medium heat. Sauté the onion, garlic, capers, and red pepper flakes until the onion is soft and a bit caramelized.

2) Add the tempeh* and sauté for about 5 to 7 minutes or until the tempeh is slightly browned.

3) Add the tomatoes, bell pepper, thyme, oregano, and vinegar. Cook for about 5 minutes, stirring occasionally or until the tomatoes start to break down and reduce. Add the olives and heat through. Season with salt and garnish with parsley, if desired.

*NOTE: *Tempeh is a high-protein soy product that is fermented with grains from the whole bean versus a processed bean. The retention of the whole bean gives tempeh a higher content of protein, dietary fiber, and vitamins.*

2 Servings

1 tablespoon **olive oil**

½ small **red onion**, thinly sliced

3 **garlic cloves**, thinly sliced

1 tablespoon **capers**

¼ teaspoon **red pepper flakes**

1 package (*8 ounces*) **tempeh**, cubed

½ cup halved **cherry tomatoes**

1 roasted **red bell pepper**, diced

1 teaspoon **dried thyme**

1 teaspoon **dried oregano**

3 teaspoons **red wine vinegar**

¼ cup chopped **green olives**

¼ cup chopped **black olives**

Sea salt

Chopped **parsley**

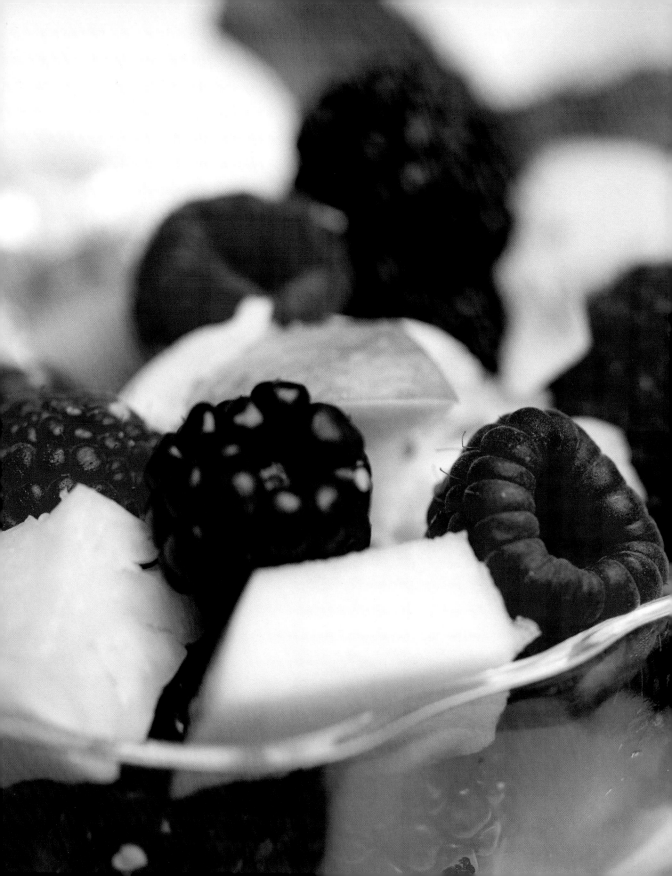

Fruit Bowl with Crème Sauce

Using any variation of fruit that is in season makes this delicious combination feel almost like a decadent dessert. Adding flax seed provides a good dose of fiber to help with fullness and blood sugar levels.

1) Put the fruit in a large bowl.

2) Blend the cashews, coconut milk, vanilla, dates, and sea salt in a blender until creamy smooth. Drizzle over the fruit and top with the cinnamon and flax seed.

2 Servings

2 cups chopped **berries** *or* **seasonal fruit of choice**

¼ cup **raw cashews**

½ cup **coconut milk** *or* **almond milk**, unsweetened

½ teaspoon **vanilla extract**

2 to 3 **Medjool dates**, pitted

Pinch of **sea salt**

Dash of **cinnamon**

1 tablespoon **ground flax seed**, for garnish

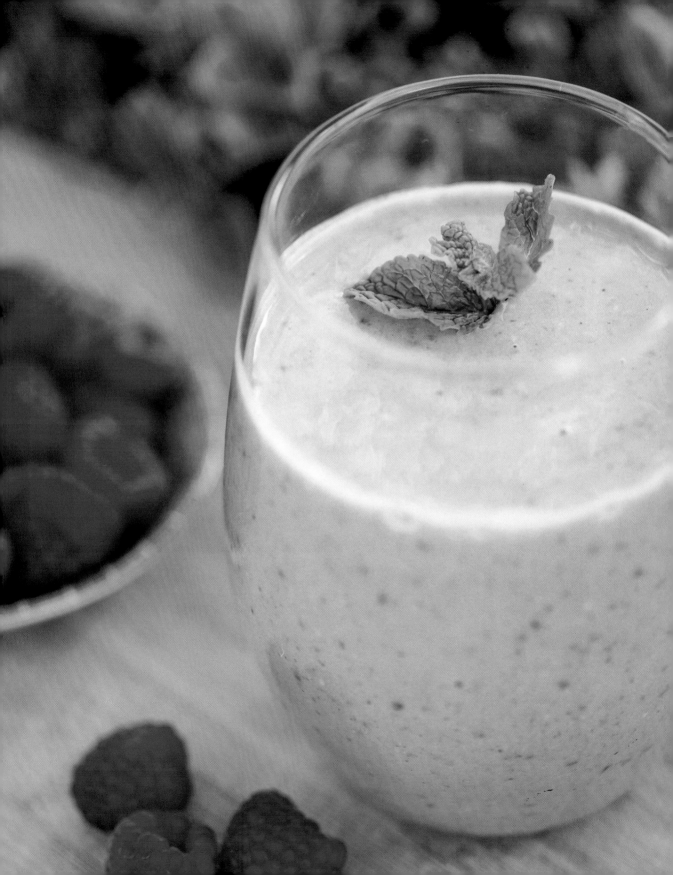

Ruby's Raspberry Dazzle Protein Shake

This simple yet delicious smoothie was created for my five-year-old sweet friend, Ruby. She loves her smoothies, and I wanted to dedicate this delicious, protein-packed delight to her.

1) Blend the ingredients in a high-powered blender until smooth and creamy.

1 Serving

1½ cups **almond milk**

½ cup **frozen raspberries**

½ **frozen banana**

½ cup **frozen strawberries**

1 scoop **vanilla protein powder**

1 tablespoon **raw almond butter**

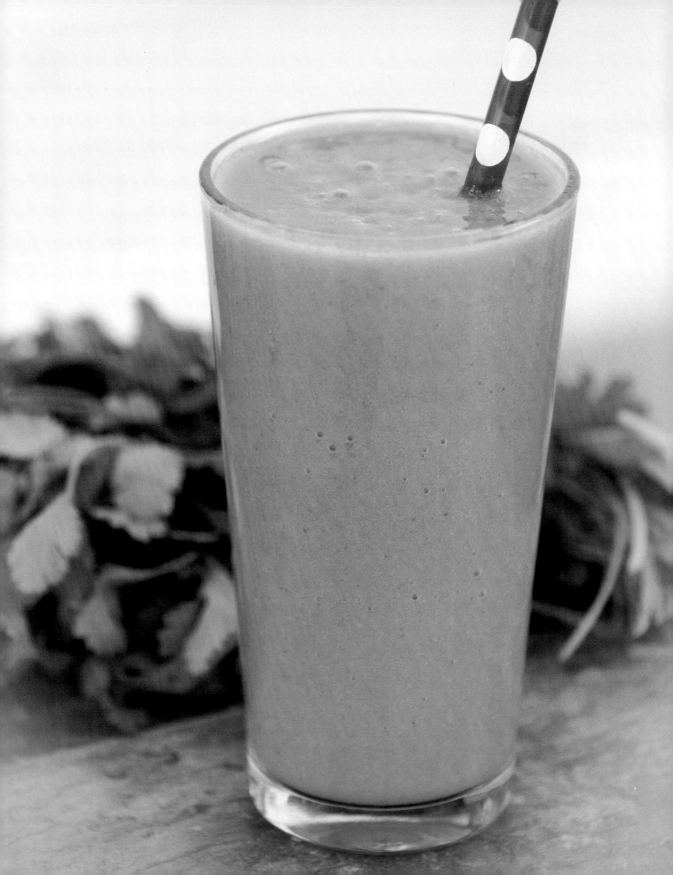

Green with Envy Smoothie*

This smoothie will help your body detox naturally using leafy greens and cilantro, which will also alkalize your system.

1) Blend the ingredients in a high-powered blender until smooth.

*NOTE: *This is a good snack option for meal plans.*

1 Serving

1½ cups **coconut water**

1 teaspoon **maca**

2 handfuls **spinach**

1 handful **kale**, any variety

1 cup **frozen mango**

½ **frozen banana**

5 **cilantro sprigs**

1 handful **ice**, optional

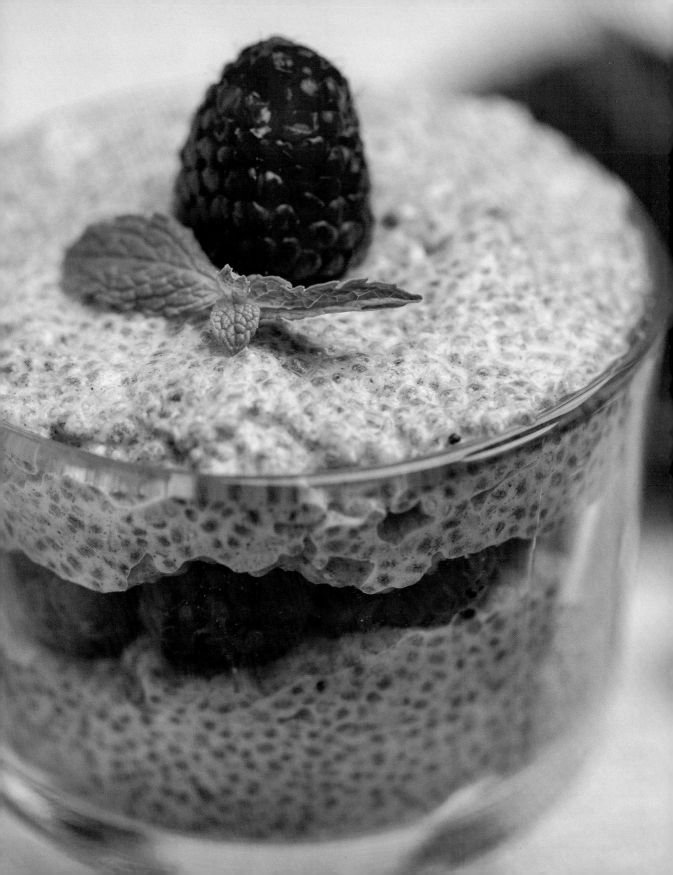

Energy Chia Breakfast Pudding*

This delicious pudding provides lots of protein, a high dose of omegas, and healthy fats for sustained energy all day. Store it tightly covered in your refrigerator and enjoy the leftovers as an afternoon or midmorning snack.

1) Put the chia seeds in a medium-sized glass or metal bowl.

2) Blend the almond or coconut milk, cashews, dates, syrup (to taste), vanilla, cinnamon, cardamom, and sea salt in a high-powered blender until creamy smooth. Pour over the chia seeds and stir well to combine.

3) Let the pudding sit for about 10 to 15 minutes, or overnight in the refrigerator, until it thickens. To serve, top with fresh raspberries or your choice of fruit and add the nuts and a splash of coconut milk, if you like.

*NOTE: *This is a good snack option for meal plans.*

2 Large Servings

½ cup whole **chia seeds**

1½ cups unsweetened **almond milk** *or* **coconut milk**

¼ cup **cashews**

2 **dates**, pitted

1 to 2 tablespoons **grade B maple syrup**

1 teaspoon **vanilla extract**

½ teaspoon **cinnamon**

¼ teaspoon **cardamom**

Pinch of **sea salt**

1 cup **fresh raspberries** *or* **other fruit in season**

Almonds *or* **any raw nuts** for topping

Gingery Miso Soup

Miso soup is superalkalizing to the system first thing in the morning. It's a ritual for the Japanese every day. The seaweed provides a good dose of iodine, which helps to strengthen your thyroid gland.

1) In a medium saucepan, bring the water, seaweed, ginger, and onion to a boil. Reduce heat and simmer for about 5 to 7 minutes. Remove from the heat.

2) In a small dish or cup, mix the miso with about 2 tablespoons of water to make a thin paste. Add this to the pan and stir well to incorporate. *Do not boil the miso!* Top with the mushrooms and serve immediately.

2 Servings

2 cups **water**

1 tablespoon **wakame seaweed**, chopped into small pieces

2 teaspoons freshly grated **ginger**

1 **green onion**, thinly sliced *(green and white parts)*

2 tablespoons **mellow white miso paste**

2 **shiitake mushrooms**, thinly sliced

Savory Brekkie Bowl

This is one of my favorite combinations to eat in the morning. Most people are used to having sweet food in the morning, but I love to have savory meals like soup or this delicious brekkie bowl, which is loaded with protein, complex carbs, and healthy fats—a fantastically savory way to start the day. Why massage the kale? Just a five-minute rubdown breaks down kale's cellulose structure, transforming this tough, bitter green to a silky and soft salad addition.

1) To massage the kale, remove the fibrous ribs, then massage the leaves with a drizzle of olive oil for a few minutes. You'll notice that as you rub the leaves, the kale will begin to change in appearance. It will become darker, shrink a bit, and become softer.

2) Once it appears "wilted," place the kale on the bottom of a bowl and top with the brown rice, hummus, and sauerkraut. Season with salt and pepper. Drizzle with dressing, if desired.

1 Serving

1 cup **raw, curly kale**, massaged

½ cup **cooked brown rice** (*kept warm*)

2 tablespoons **hummus**

¼ cup cultured, **raw sauerkraut**

Sea salt and freshly **ground pepper**

Dressing of your choice (*optional*)

Other Shakes, Teas, and Comfort Treats

These shakes, elixirs, and teas
can be made throughout the cleanse
as either a snack or a special,
comforting treat.

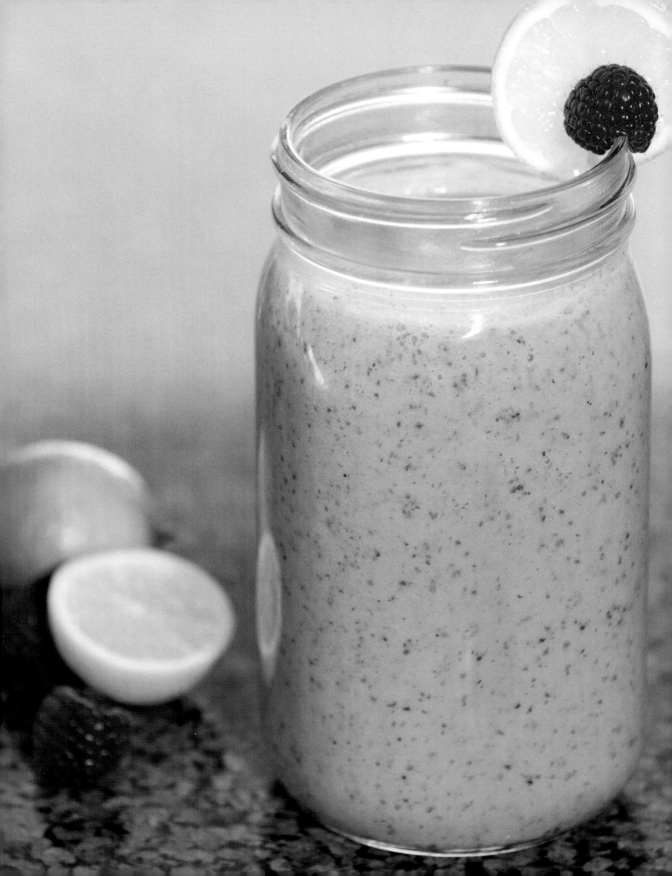

Pear Cilantro Shake*

This shake is a great detoxifier. The cilantro helps to cleanse any heavy metals from your body, as well as providing a fresh, snappy flavor. Adding avocado provides a healthy dose of good fats, which your body needs and utilizes for energy.

1) Blend the ingredients in a high-powered blender until smooth.

*NOTE: *This is a good snack option for meal plans.*

1 Serving

- 1 **ripe pear**, cored
- 1¼ cups unsweetened **coconut water** *or* **almond milk**
- 1 handful **fresh cilantro**
- ¼ **avocado**
- 2 teaspoons **lime juice**
- 2 teaspoons **maple syrup**
- 1 handful **ice** *(optional)*

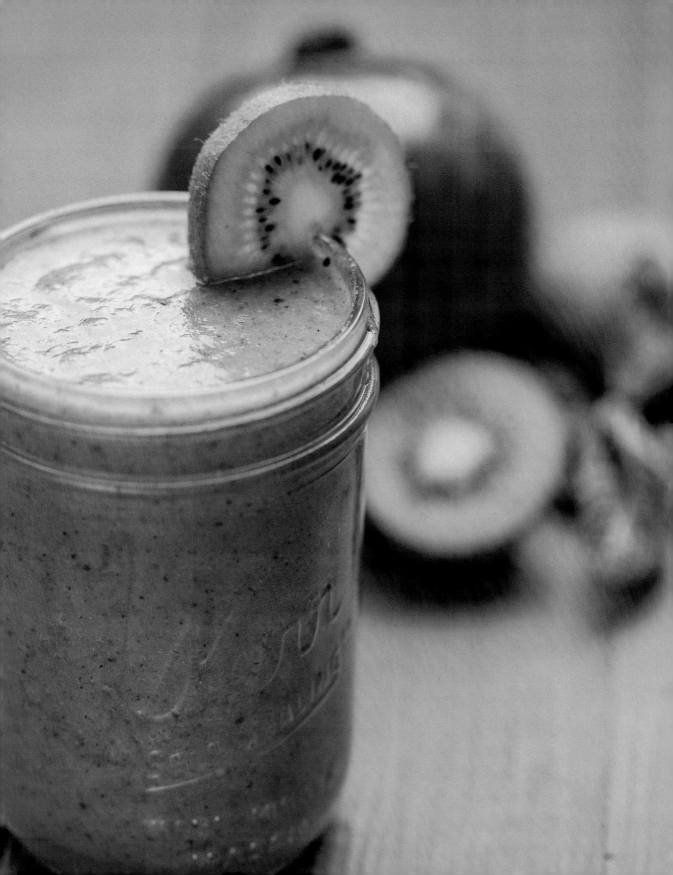

Pineapple Minty Refresher*

Pineapple with mint is one of my favorite combinations.
This delicious shake will help to heal your digestive tract.

1) Blend the ingredients in a high-powered blender until smooth. If it is too thick, add more coconut water while blending.

*NOTE: *This is a good snack option for meal plans.*

1 Serving

- 1¼ cups **coconut water**
- 1 cup frozen **pineapple**
- ½ cup chopped **honeydew** *or* ½ cup **seedless red** *or* **green grapes**
- 10 leaves **fresh mint**
- 1 **whole kiwi**, skin removed
- 1 handful **curly kale** *or* **romaine leaves** *(kale will result in a stronger flavor)*
- ¼ teaspoon **coriander**
- 1 handful **ice** *(optional)*

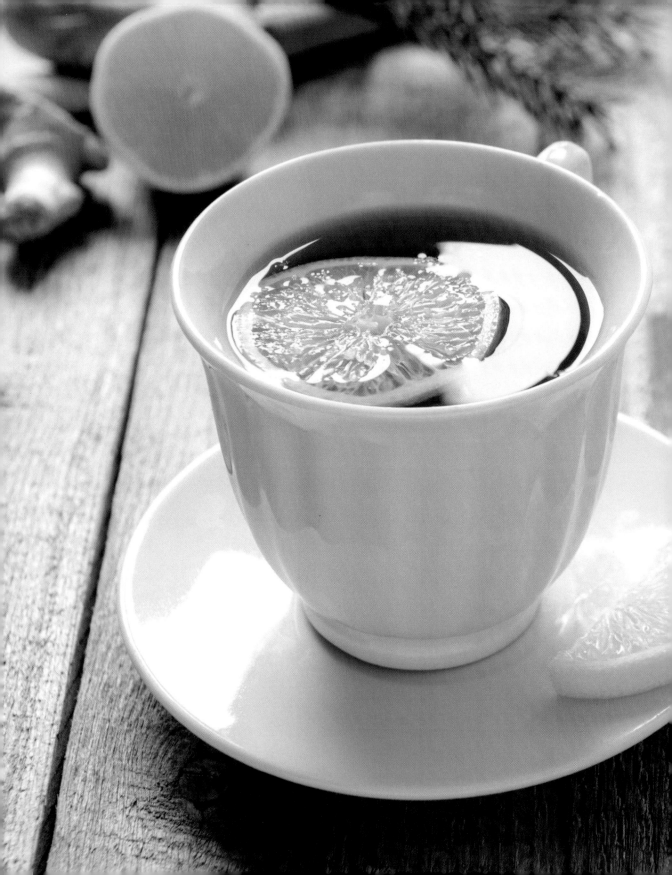

AI Tea *(Anti-Inflammatory Tea)*

This tea is great for helping joint pain, as well as digestive issues. It's great served hot or as an iced tea, and can be sipped after meals to support digestion.

1) Put the water, ginger, and turmeric root in a saucepan and bring to a boil. Turn the heat to low and simmer for about 20 minutes.

2) Strain tea into a pitcher or jar. Add lemon juice and sweetener to taste.

Four 8-ounce Servings

4 cups filtered **water**

3-inch piece **ginger**, peeled and thinly sliced

3-inch piece fresh **turmeric root**, peeled and thinly sliced *or* 2 teaspoons **powdered turmeric**

Juice of 2 medium **lemons** *(about ⅓ to ½ cup)*

Raw honey *or* **stevia**

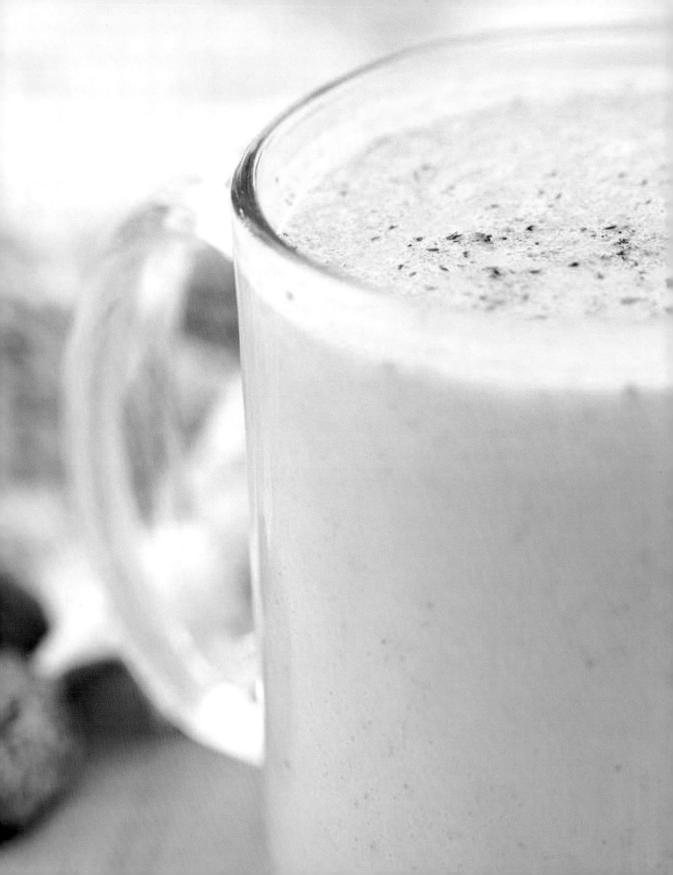

Creamy Golden Milk

Here is an amazing Ayurvedic remedy for achy joints and rheumatoid arthritis, and it's delicious too. This is my own version with the addition of ginger, which helps to cool inflammation and aid digestion.

1) Heat the oil in a small saucepan until melted.

2) Add the turmeric and ginger, and sizzle for 30 seconds.

3) Add the almond milk to the saucepan and heat just before boiling. Sweeten with honey or maple syrup and top with a dash of nutmeg.

1 Serving

2 teaspoons **coconut oil**

½ teaspoon **powdered turmeric**

¼ teaspoon **powdered ginger**

1 cup unsweetened **almond milk**

Raw honey *or* **maple syrup** to taste

Dash of **nutmeg**

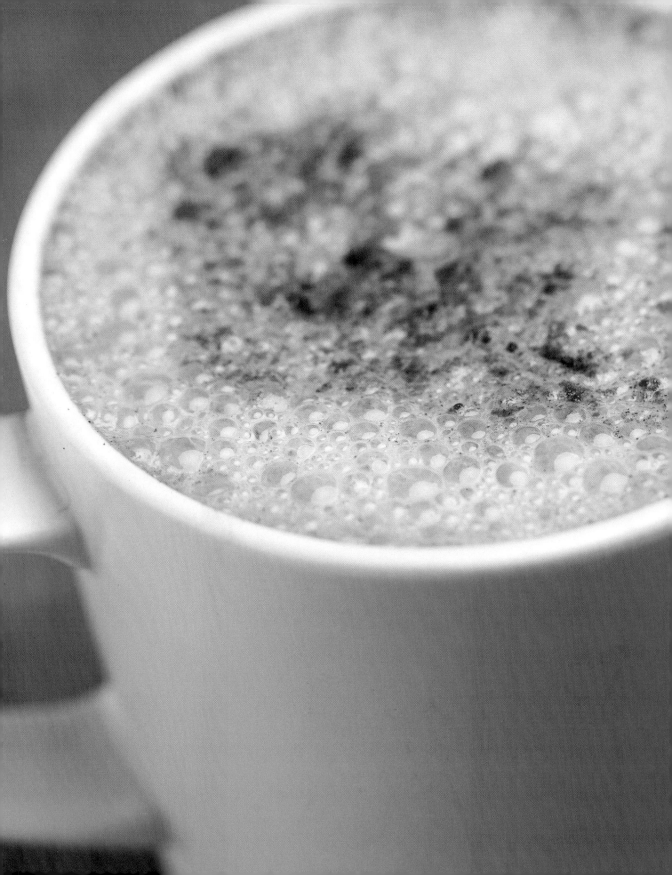

Spiced Almond Milk

Nighttime sugar cravings got ahold of you? Try this luscious and creamy warmed almond milk to satisfy those cravings in a healthy way—awesome right before bed to soothe you to sleep!

1) Whisk the ingredients together in a saucepan and heat gently over low heat until warm.

1 Serving

10 to 12 ounces unsweetened **almond milk**

½ teaspoon **vanilla extract**

4 drops **stevia** *or* 2 teaspoons **maple syrup**

Dash of **nutmeg**

½ teaspoon **cinnamon**

Dash of **cloves**

Snazzy and Satisfying Salads

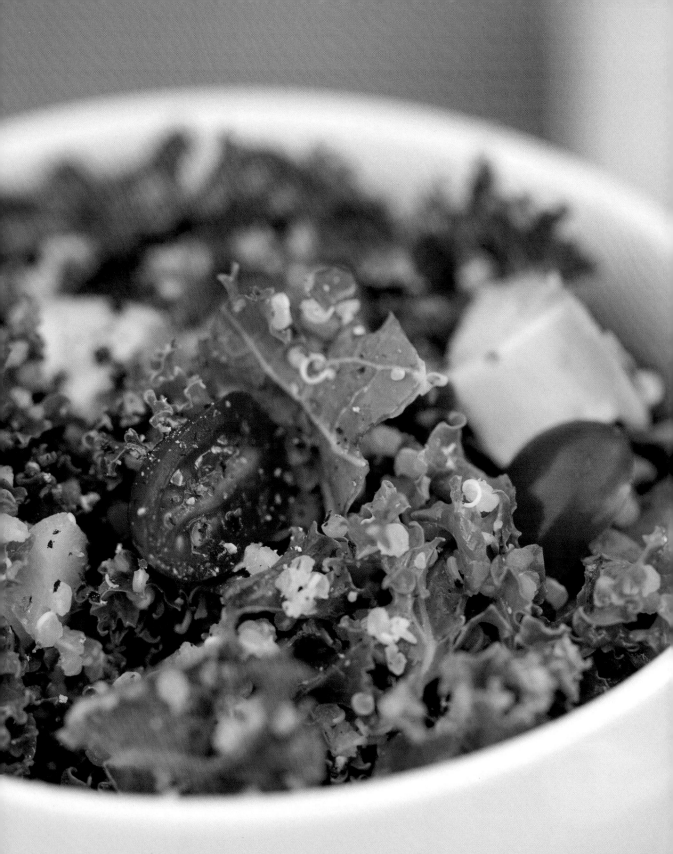

Kale and Quinoa Power Salad

This power-packed salad pairs high-protein quinoa with chlorophyll-rich kale. This nutrient-rich combo will alkalize your body and help to detoxify your kidneys and liver too.

1) Put the kale, quinoa, avocado, tomatoes, onion, and seeds in a bowl.

2) In a separate bowl, whisk the lemon juice and oil together. Pour over the salad and toss until well mixed. Season with salt and pepper.

2 Servings

3 cups **curly kale**, de-stemmed and torn into bite-size pieces

1 cup cooked **quinoa**

½ **avocado**, cubed

¼ cup **cherry tomatoes**, halved

2 tablespoons diced **red onion**

2 tablespoons **hemp seeds**

Juice of 2 medium **lemons** (*about ⅓ to ½ cup*)

2 tablespoons **olive oil**

Sea salt and **pepper**

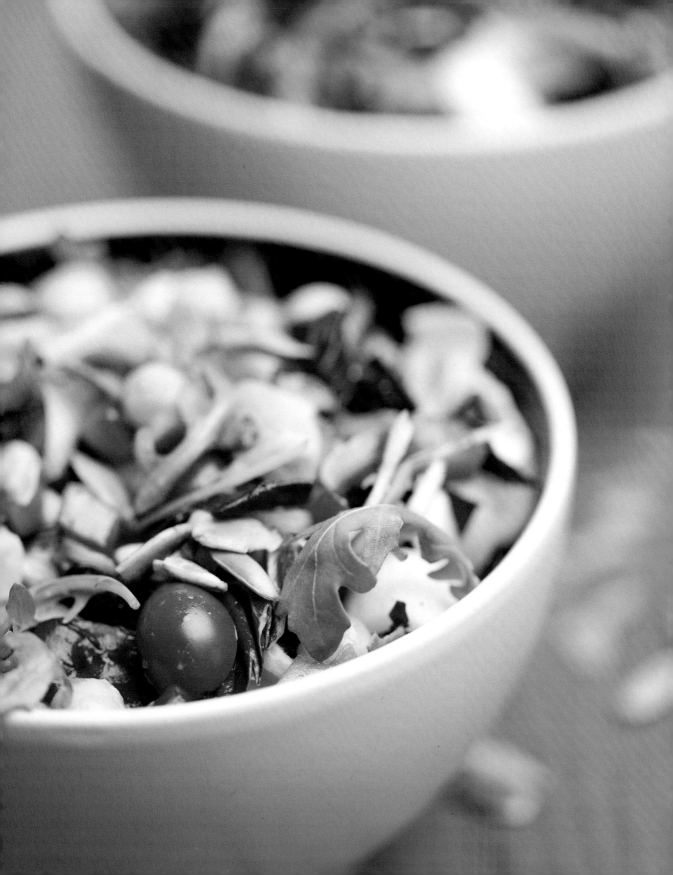

Chopped Salad with Shallot Vinaigrette

The bitter greens in this salad will help detoxify your major organs. Chickpeas add protein, and avocado adds skin-glowing, healthy fats—a satisfying and delicious combo!

1) Combine the salad ingredients in a large bowl.

2) Blend the vinaigrette ingredients in a blender or shake in a shaker bottle until well mixed. Toss the salad greens with the vinaigrette and serve.

2 Servings

Salad:

2 heads endive, finely chopped

½ small head radicchio, finely chopped

1 cup arugula

½ cup cooked chickpeas

¼ cup pitted kalamata olives, roughly chopped

½ orange or red bell pepper, deseeded and diced

¼ avocado, cubed

½ cup cherry tomatoes, halved

¼ cup finely diced red onion

¼ cup toasted pumpkin seeds

Sea salt and pepper

Shallot Vinaigrette:

1 shallot, minced

1 tablespoon Dijon mustard

2 teaspoons maple syrup or 3 drops stevia liquid (optional)

¼ cup olive oil

⅓ cup rice wine vinegar

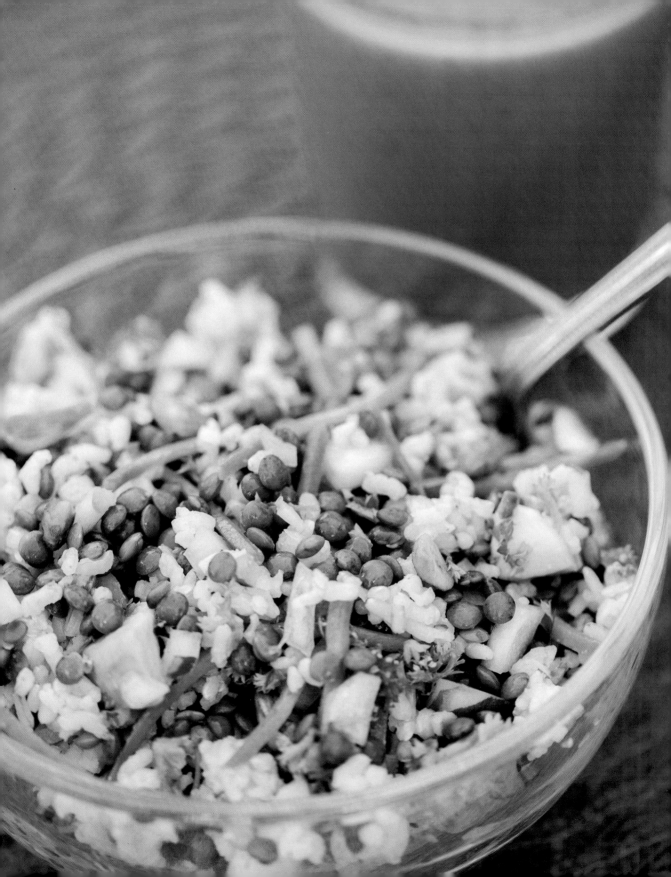

Herbed Brown Rice and Lentil Salad with Lime Dressing

Lentils and brown rice combined make this salad high in fiber, protein and complex carbs. It's an awesome dish that will keep you satisfied and your blood sugar balanced during the day.

1) Put the salad ingredients in a large bowl.

2) Blend the dressing ingredients in a blender until smooth and pour on the salad. Toss until well mixed.

2 Servings

Salad:

1 cup cooked brown rice

1 cup cooked Puy lentils

¼ cup diced red onion

¼ cup grated *or* shredded carrots

½ avocado, cubed

¼ cup pistachios

¼ cup freshly chopped parsley

Sea salt and fresh cracked pepper

Lime Dressing:

2 garlic cloves

Juice of 2 medium limes *(about 3 to 4 tablespoons)*

2 tablespoons sesame oil

3 tablespoons unsweetened rice vinegar

Drizzle of maple syrup

Sea salt

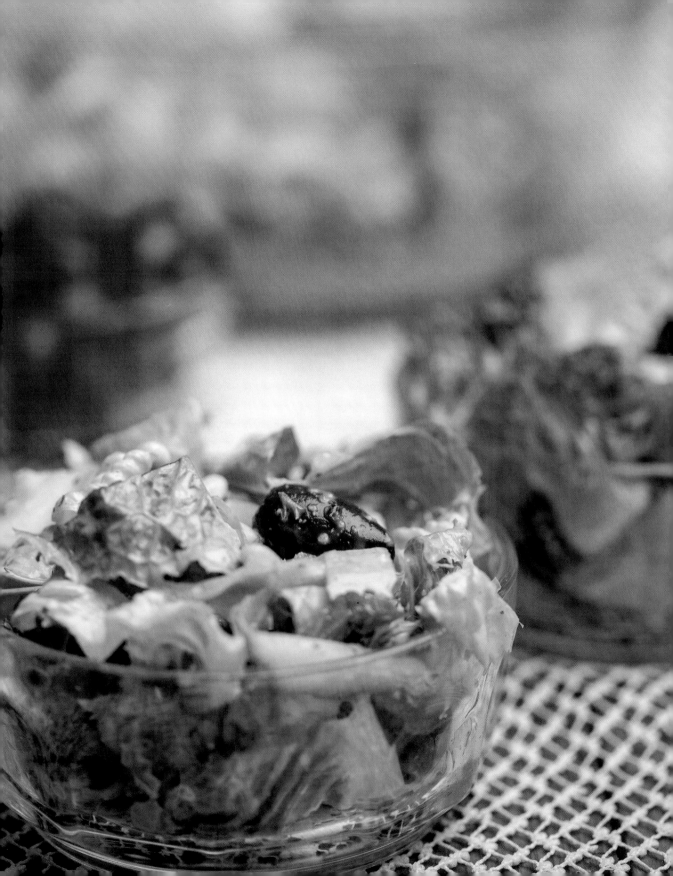

Gracious Greek Salad

Who doesn't love Greek salad? This dairy-free version is a delight and loaded with phytonutrients, fat dissolvers, and antioxidants.

1) Put the salad ingredients in a large salad bowl.

2) Blend the dressing ingredients in a blender until creamy smooth. Pour over the salad and toss until well mixed.

2 Servings

Salad:

3 cups chopped romaine lettuce

¼ cup chopped cucumber

½ red bell pepper, diced

¼ cup chopped kalamata olives

¼ cup cherry tomatoes, halved

2 tablespoons capers, drained

2 tablespoons diced red onion

2 tablespoons chopped parsley

Garlicky Greek Dressing:

¼ cup olive oil

2 tablespoons apple cider vinegar

1 tablespoon hemp seeds

2 garlic cloves

1 tablespoon lemon juice

1 teaspoon dried oregano

2 teaspoons Dijon mustard

3 teaspoons maple syrup

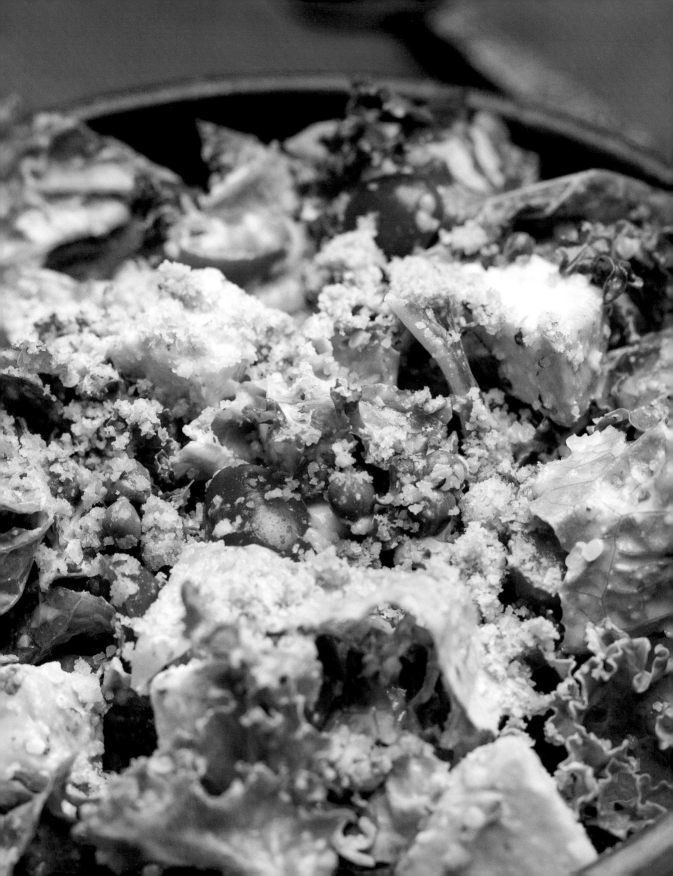

Creamy Kale and Avocado Caesar with "Cheese" Sprinkles

1) Put the salad ingredients in a bowl.

2) Blend the dressing ingredients in a blender until creamy smooth. Pour the dressing over the salad and toss until well mixed. Top with "Cheese" Sprinkles.

2 Servings

Salad:

3 cups curly kale, torn into bite-size pieces

1 cup chopped romaine lettuce

½ cup cherry tomatoes, halved

2 tablespoons hemp seeds

¼ avocado, cubed

1 tablespoon capers

Pumpkin Seed Caesar Dressing:

2 tablespoons apple cider vinegar

¼ cup lightly toasted pumpkin seeds

3 tablespoons nutritional yeast

2 teaspoons Dijon mustard

2 tablespoons lemon juice

1 tablespoon maple syrup

¼ cup extra virgin olive oil

1 garlic clove

½ teaspoon sea salt

Freshly ground pepper (optional)

"Cheese" Sprinkles

1) Grind the nuts with the yeast and salt in a blender or coffee grinder.

6 Servings

½ cup lightly toasted walnuts

3 tablespoons nutritional yeast

¼ teaspoon sea salt

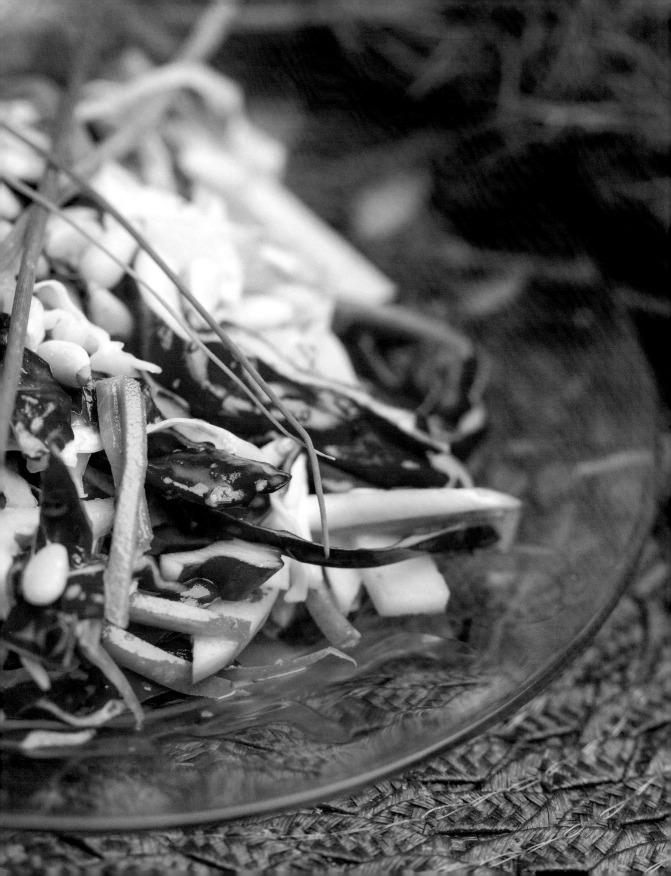

Snappy Slaw with Lime Cilantro Vinaigrette

This snappy version of everyday coleslaw includes fat-emulsifying daikon radish. Cabbage is one of the best foods to eat for cancer prevention and also helps eliminate toxins from your system.

1) Put the salad ingredients in a large bowl.

2) Blend the vinaigrette ingredients in a blender and puree until smooth. Pour the vinaigrette over the salad and toss until well mixed.

2 Servings

Salad:

1 cup shredded **red cabbage**

1 cup shredded **green** or **Napa cabbage**

½ cup shredded **carrots**

½ cup shredded **green apple** with skin

¼ cup grated **daikon radish**

Lime Cilantro Vinaigrette:

1 large handful **cilantro leaves**

¼ cup **extra virgin olive oil**

¼ cup freshly squeezed **lime juice**

1 **garlic** clove, minced

1 tablespoon **grade B maple syrup**

2 tablespoons **rice vinegar** (*unseasoned*)

¼ teaspoon **sea salt**

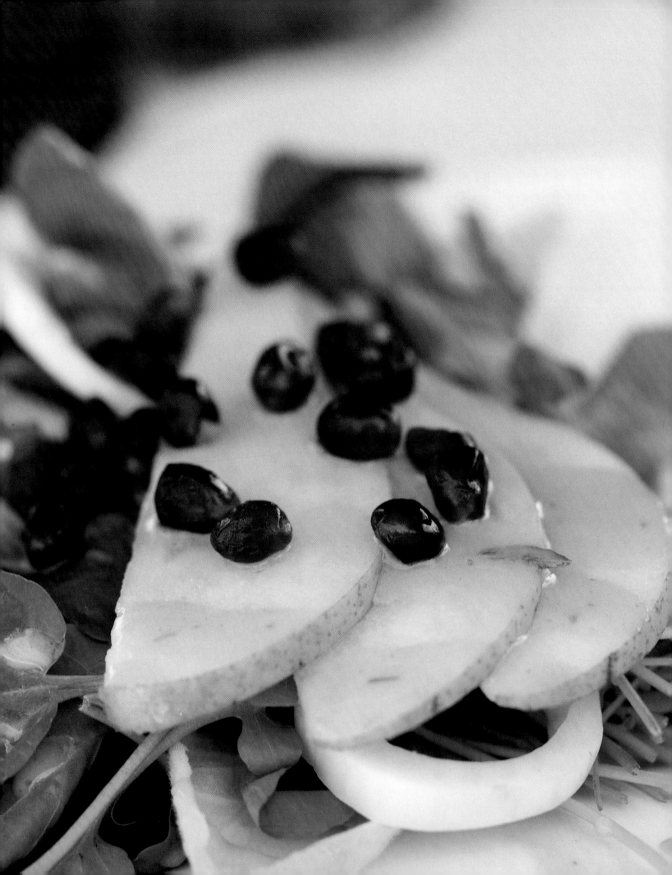

Watercress, Pear, and Fennel Salad with Tarragon Vinaigrette

Fennel is a phenomenal digestive aid, and watercress is great for flushing the kidneys. Fresh tarragon in the dressing gives this delicious salad an herby touch.

1) Put the salad ingredients in a large bowl.

2) In a separate bowl, whisk together the vinaigrette ingredients. Drizzle the vinaigrette over the salad and toss to coat.

2 Servings

Salad:

1 bunch of watercress *(about 2 cups)*

1 head endive, finely chopped

¼ cup thinly sliced fennel

1 ripe pear, cored and thinly sliced

2 tablespoons pine nuts

Tarragon Vinaigrette:

1 teaspoon dried tarragon

2 teaspoons Dijon mustard

3 tablespoons apple cider vinegar

4 tablespoons olive oil

Dash of maple syrup

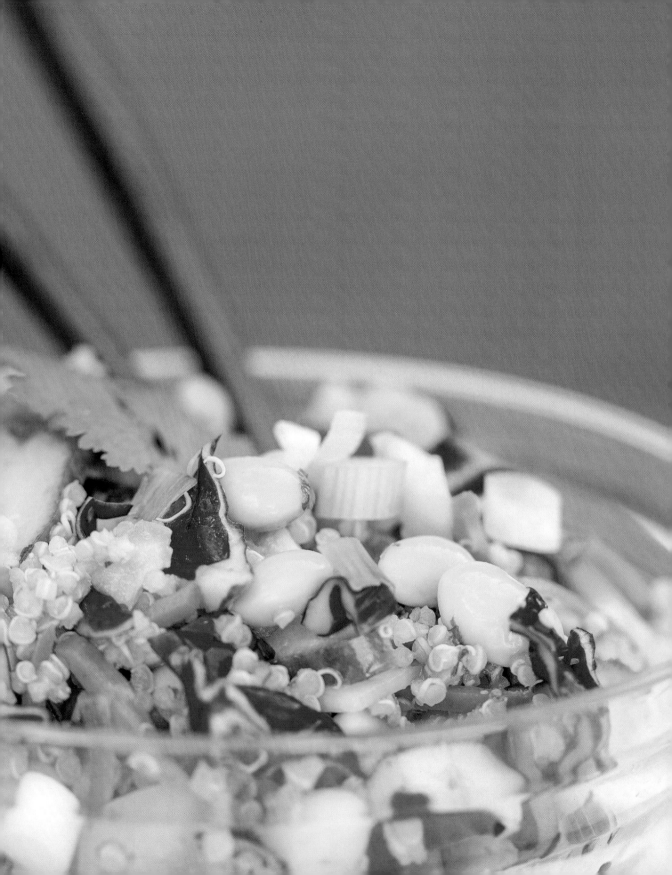

Asian-Style Quinoa Salad

A high-protein combination of edamame beans and quinoa in this Asian salad will leave you feeling satisfied. High-antioxidant peppers and cabbage are great detoxifiers as well.

1) Put the salad ingredients in a large bowl.

2) Whisk the dressing ingredients together in a small bowl. Toss the salad with the dressing and let it sit for 5 to 10 minutes so all the flavors are incorporated.

2 to 3 Servings

Salad:

1 cup shelled edamame beans, cooked according to package directions

1 cup cooked quinoa

½ cup diced cucumber (*about one-half medium cucumber*)

¼ cup diced yellow *or* red bell pepper

1 cup chopped red cabbage

¼ cup shredded carrots

2 tablespoons sesame seeds

Asian Dressing:

3 tablespoons Bragg's Liquid Aminos

1 tablespoon sesame oil

2 tablespoons rice vinegar

2 tablespoons chopped green onion

¼ cup finely chopped cilantro

2 teaspoons maple syrup

Pinch of red pepper flakes

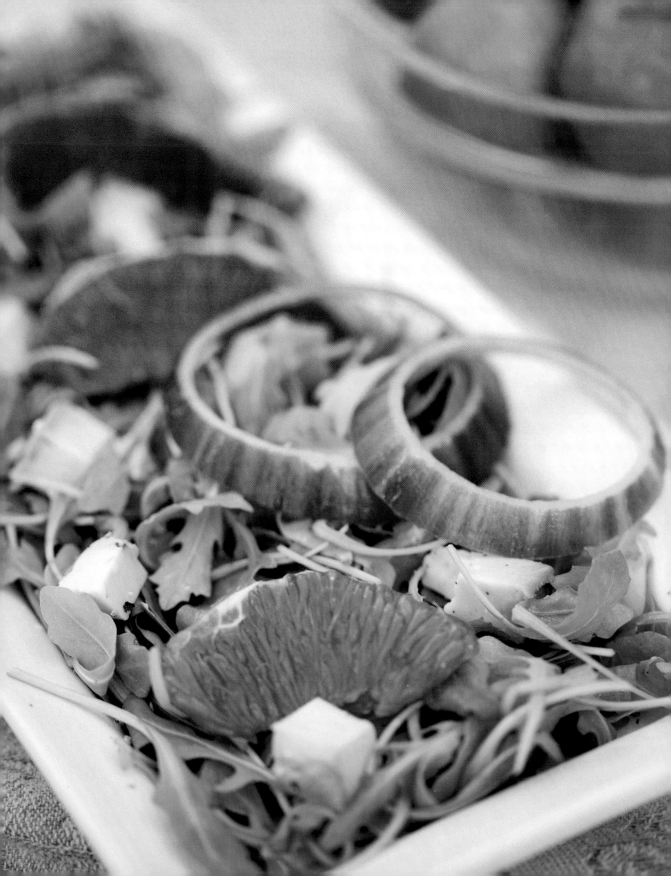

Grapefruit, Avocado, and Arugula Salad with Citrus Dressing

Fat-burning grapefruit and peppery, detoxifying arugula are perfect paired with skin-glowing avocado in this delicious salad that packs a citrus punch.

1) Put the salad ingredients in a large bowl.

2) Blend the dressing ingredients in a blender or shake them in a shaker bottle until well combined. Pour the dressing over the salad and toss until well mixed.

2 Servings

Salad:

1 large Ruby Red grapefruit, peeled and sectioned

½ avocado, cubed

4 cups arugula

¼ cup thinly sliced red onion

Sea salt and pepper

Citrus Dressing:

Juice of 1 medium orange *(about 3 tablespoons)*

Juice of 1 medium lime *(about 2 tablespoons)*

1 tablespoon Bragg's Liquid Aminos *or* low-sodium soy sauce

1 tablespoon maple syrup

2 tablespoons sesame oil

3 tablespoons unsweetened rice vinegar

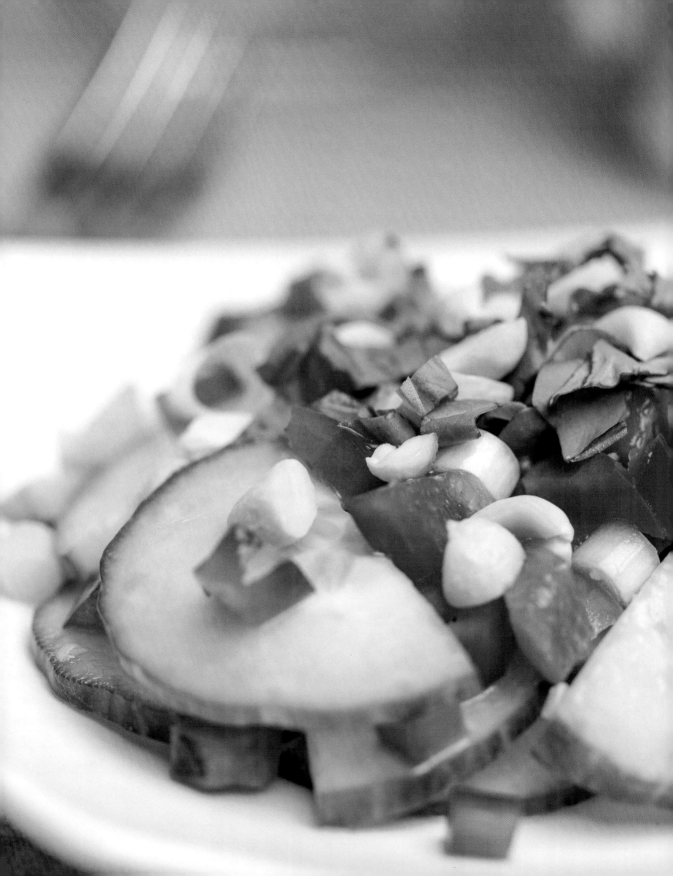

Thai Cucumber Salad with Lime Dressing

Cucumbers have a high water content, making them perfect for flushing and detoxifying the system. This Thai-style salad is full of flavor and nutrients.

1) Put the salad ingredients in a medium-sized bowl.

2) In a separate bowl, whisk together the dressing ingredients. Pour the dressing over the salad and toss well to combine.

2 Servings

Salad:

1 English cucumber, halved lengthwise and cut into ¼-inch-wide half rounds

½ yellow or red bell pepper, deseeded and diced small

2 scallions, finely chopped

2 tablespoons freshly chopped basil

2 tablespoons chopped cashews or peanuts

Lime Dressing:

Juice of 1 medium lime (about 2 tablespoons)

1 garlic clove, minced

1 tablespoon Bragg's Liquid Aminos

1 tablespoon rice vinegar

2 tablespoons sesame oil

1 tablespoon water

Pinch of red pepper flakes

2 to 4 drops stevia or 1 tablespoon maple syrup

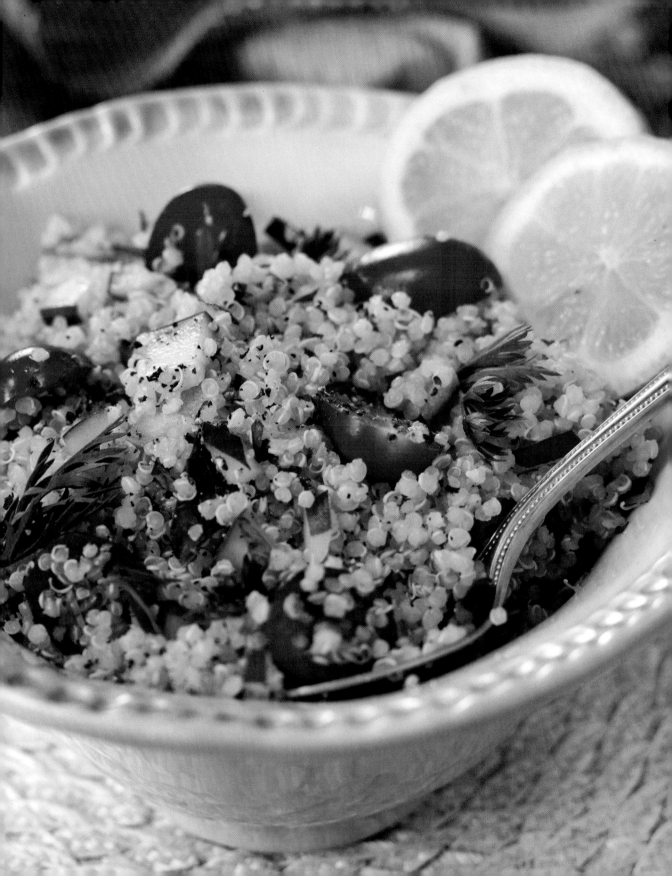

Quinoa Tabbouleh Salad

High-protein, gluten-free quinoa replaces bulgur wheat in this traditional Mediterranean salad. It's great as a side dish or tossed on top of a green salad to add an extra punch of nutrients.

1) Cook the quinoa according to package directions.

2) Once cooked, transfer to a large bowl to cool. Add the remaining ingredients and stir to combine. Season with salt and pepper to taste.

4 to 6 Servings

1 cup **quinoa**

2 cups **water**

½ cup chopped **fresh mint**

½ cup chopped **fresh parsley**

1 small **cucumber**, peeled and diced (*about 1 cup*)

1 cup **cherry tomatoes**, halved

2 tablespoons **olive oil**

2 **garlic cloves**, minced

¼ cup **lemon juice**

Sea salt and **pepper**

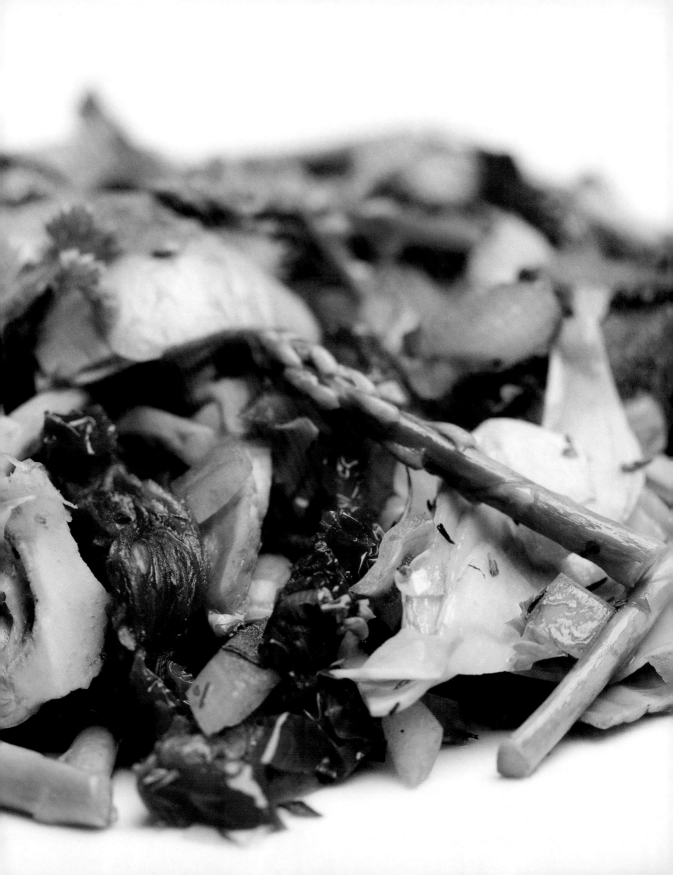

Warmed Wild Mushroom and Asparagus Salad

Shiitake mushrooms have intense healing powers. Paired with kidney-cleansing artichokes and asparagus, this dish is a powerhouse of detoxifying goodness.

1) Heat the oil in a medium-sized skillet over medium heat and sauté the onion and mushrooms. Add the asparagus, artichoke hearts, tomatoes, thyme, vinegar, and water. Cover with a lid and cook for about 5 to 7 minutes or until the asparagus is tender and the artichoke hearts are warmed through.

3 Servings

1 tablespoon olive oil

1 small yellow onion, diced (about ½ cup)

6 shiitake mushrooms, thinly sliced

½ bunch of asparagus (about 8–10 stalks), woody ends removed and cut into ½-inch pieces

1 cup rinsed and roughly chopped artichoke hearts (canned or jarred)

4 sundried tomatoes, presoaked in warm water, drained, and cut into small strips

1 teaspoon dried thyme

2 tablespoons balsamic vinegar

2 tablespoons water

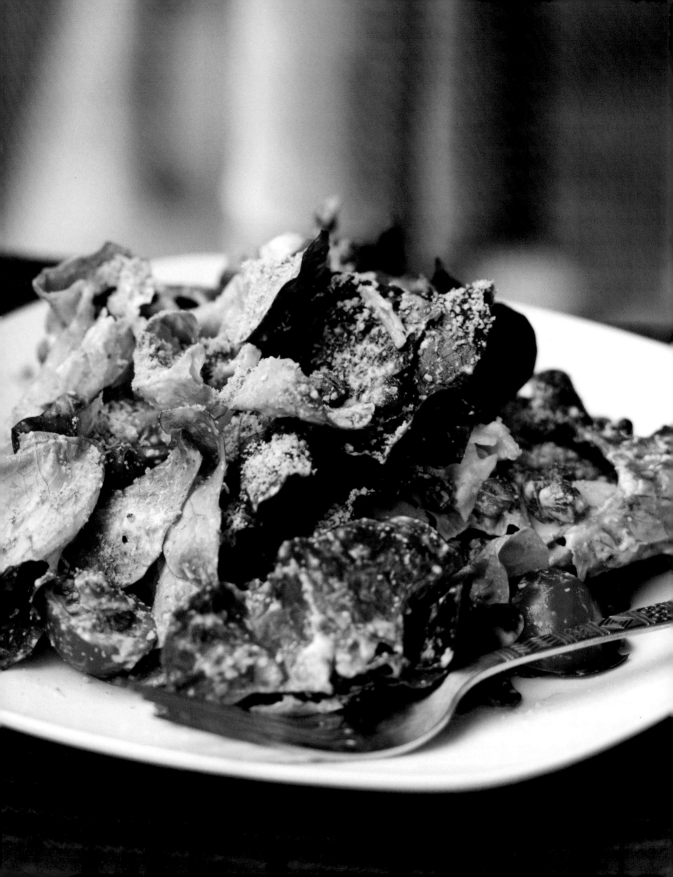

Salad of Your Choice . . .

Whenever you see "salad of your choice" noted in the meal plans, refer to this page to help you construct a sassy and succulent salad. Be creative and turn your salads into a hearty meal. My favorite light and delicious dressing on a salad is a drizzle of olive oil or walnut oil with a squeeze of lemon and a pinch of sea salt. This combo helps to pop the flavor of the salad without overpowering it.

Greens

Arugula

Baby greens

Dandelion greens

Endive

Escarole

Kale

Mesclun mix

Radicchio

Spinach

Sprouts

Swiss chard

Proteins

Beans *(any)*

Nuts and seeds *(any raw)*

Tempeh

Veggies

Artichoke hearts

Beets *(shredded)*

Bell peppers

Broccoli

Butternut squash, cubed

Cabbage *(shredded)*

Carrots *(shredded)*

Cauliflower

Celery

Corn *(raw)*

Cucumbers

Fennel

Hearts of palm

Mushrooms

Radishes

Tomatoes

Yams *(diced and cooked)*

Grains

Amaranth

Brown rice

Buckwheat

Millet

Quinoa

Wild rice

Fruits

Avocado

Blueberries

Dried fruit *(minimal and no sugar added)*

Grapes

Olives

Peaches

Strawberries

Tomatoes

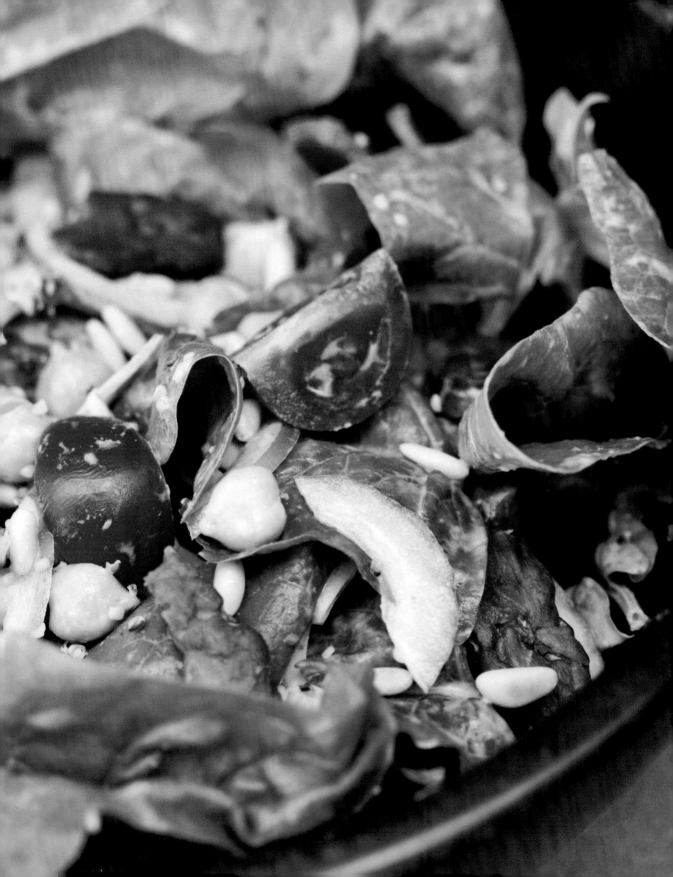

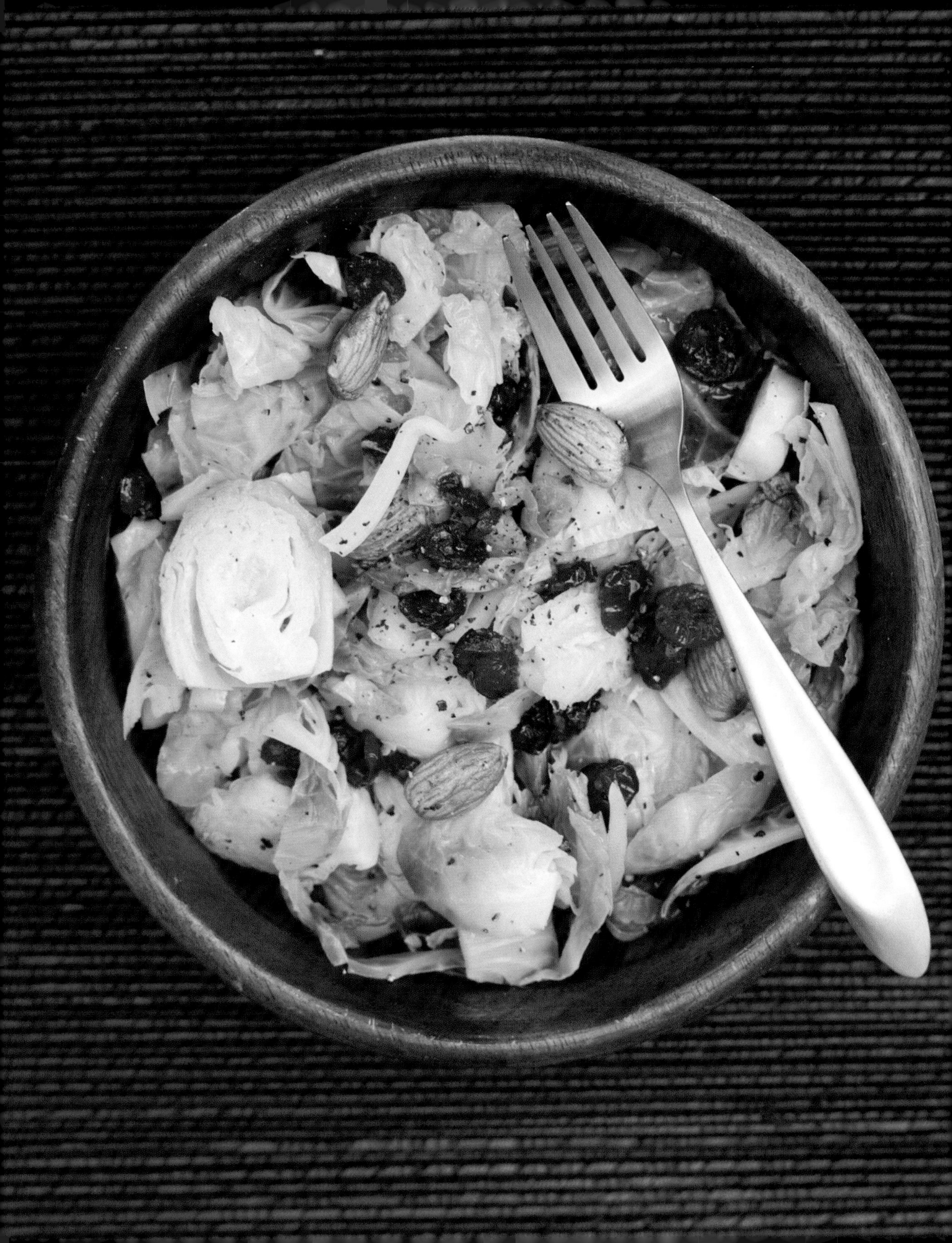

Slurp–Worthy Soups and Stews

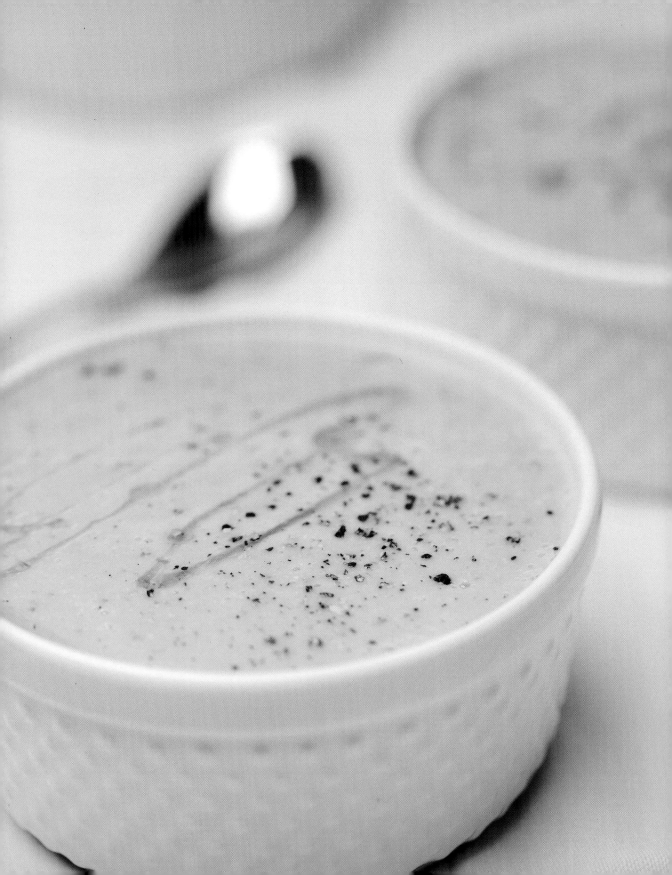

Sweet Pea Soup

Fiber-rich sweet peas make this surprisingly delicious and simple soup filling and satisfying. The mint will aid your digestion, as well as add a fresh zing.

1) Heat the oil in a large saucepan over medium heat. Add the leek, scallions, and garlic, and sauté for 5 minutes. Add the broth and peas. Bring to a simmer for about 10 minutes.

2) Remove from the heat and add the lime juice, and mint.

3) Puree the soup with the cashews in a blender until creamy. Season with salt and pepper to taste.

4 Servings

1 tablespoon coconut oil

1 small leek, white parts thinly sliced

3 scallions, thinly sliced

2 garlic cloves, minced

3 cups low-sodium vegetable broth

3 cups fresh or frozen sweet peas

Juice of ½ medium lime (about 1 tablespoon)

2 tablespoons fresh mint, finely chopped

½ cup cashews, soaked for 20 minutes

Sea salt and pepper

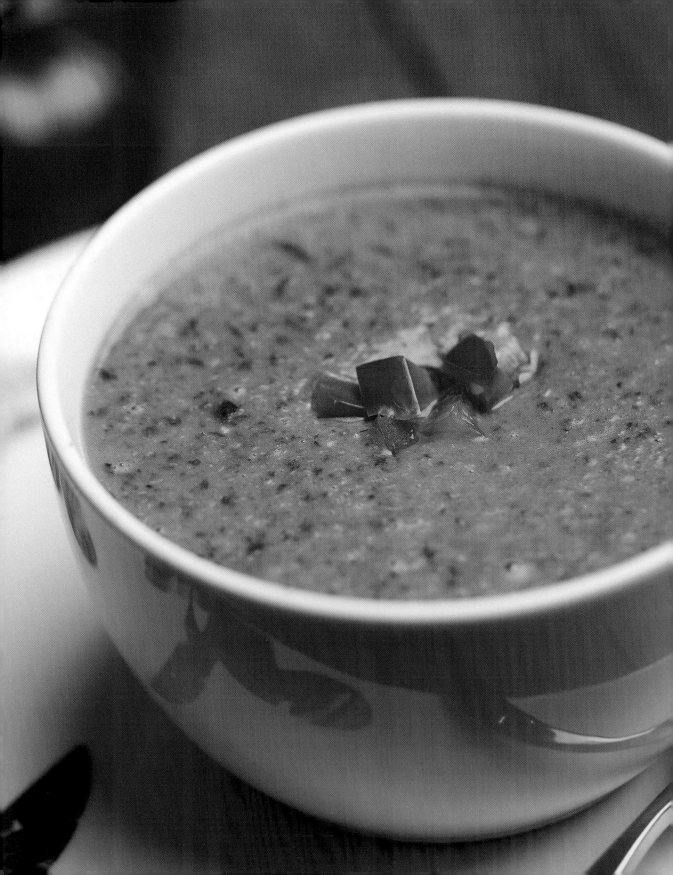

Caribbean Black Bean Soup

This tropical take on black bean soup pairs potassium-rich bananas with fiber-rich black beans for a taste of the Caribbean. Black beans aid our digestive tract by producing butyric acid, which is the primary energy source for colonic cells.

1) Heat the oil in a soup pot over medium heat. Sauté the onion, garlic, and pepper until soft.

2) Add the cumin, ginger, and cayenne, if using, and stir to combine. Add the bananas, black beans, and vegetable broth. Bring to a boil, cover, turn down the heat, and simmer about 20 minutes until the fruit is soft.

3) Add the coconut milk and then puree using a blender or stick blender. Season with salt.

4 Servings

1 tablespoon coconut oil

1 small red onion, diced (about ½ cup)

2 garlic cloves, minced

1 large red bell pepper, diced (about 1 cup)

2 teaspoons cumin

1 teaspoon ground ginger

⅛ teaspoon cayenne pepper (optional)

2 large ripe bananas, sliced

3 cups black beans, drained and rinsed (about 2 cans)

3 cups vegetable broth

½ cup canned coconut milk

Sea salt

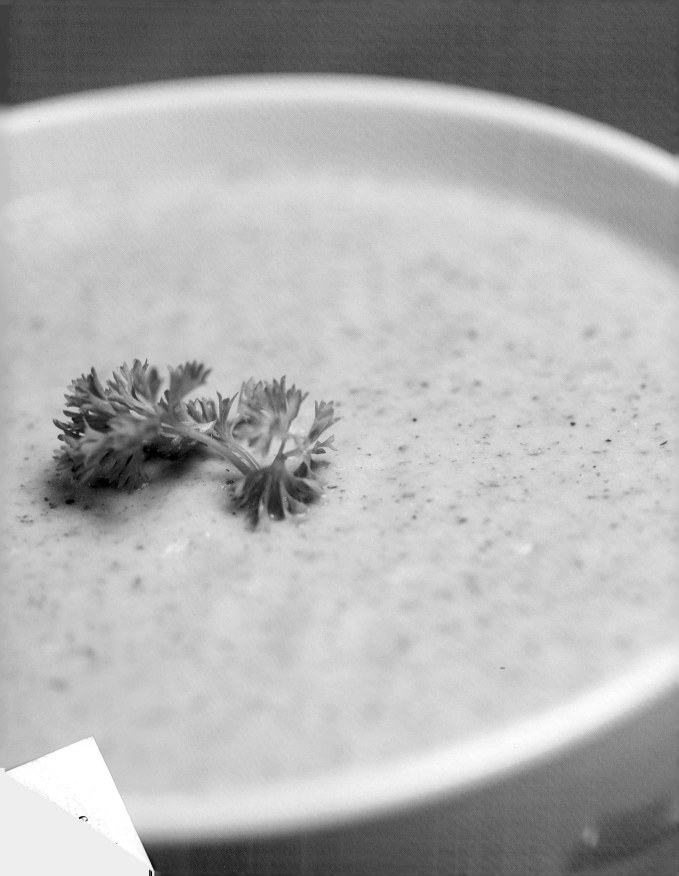

Gregarious Green Soup

Chlorophyll-rich veggies combined in a delicious and detoxifying soup will satisfy you and cleanse your body at the same time. It's gregariously good!

1) Steam the zucchini, green beans, broccoli, onion, potatoes, garlic, and spinach until slightly soft and the veggies are bright green.

2) Place the veggies in a blender with the steam water, parsley, dill, cayenne, cashews, and lime juice. Season with the sea salt or Bragg's to taste. Blend on high until creamy smooth. Add more water if needed. Top with the fresh cracked pepper.

2 to 3 Servings

1 large zucchini, chopped

1½ cups green beans, cut into 1-inch pieces

1 cup broccoli florets

¼ cup chopped onion

2 small red potatoes, cut into ¼-inch cubes

2 garlic cloves

1 handful spinach

1 handful fresh parsley

1 handful fresh dill or cilantro

Dash of cayenne pepper

⅓ cup cashews

Juice from ½ medium lime
(about 1 tablespoon)

Sea salt

Bragg's Liquid Aminos

Fresh cracked pepper

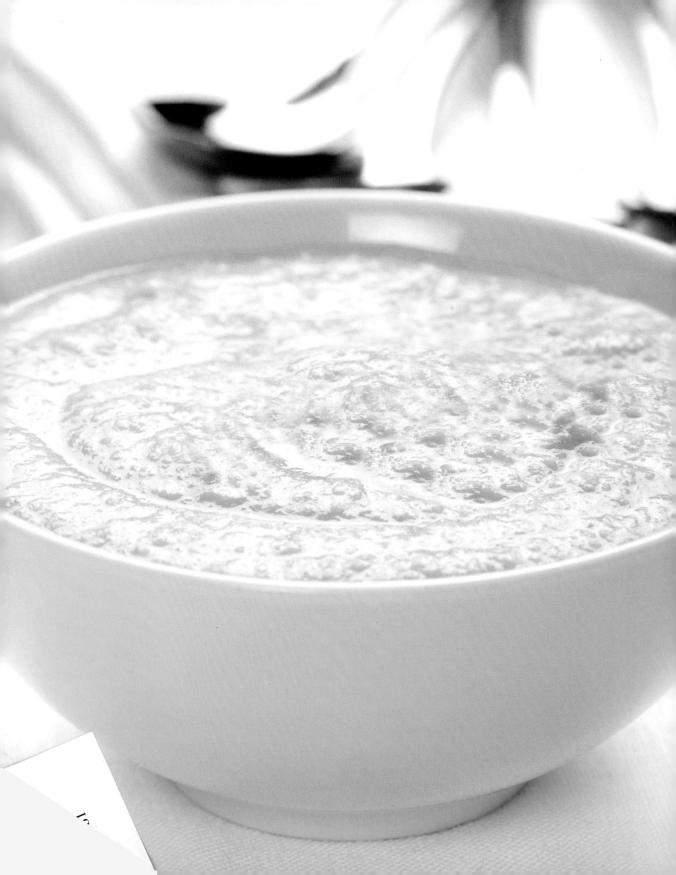

White Bean and Thyme Soup

This soup is loaded with fiber and flavor. Eating beans regularly can reduce your risk of coronary artery disease as well as keep your colon healthy and happy. They are also great for balancing blood sugar throughout the day.

1) Heat the oil over medium heat in a large soup pot. Sauté the onions and garlic until soft. Add the beans, potatoes, broth, and thyme. Turn the heat to high, bring to a boil, cover the pot, and reduce the heat to a simmer. Simmer until the potatoes are soft.

2) Puree the soup using a hand blender or regular blender.

4 Servings

1 tablespoon olive oil

1 medium yellow onion, diced

2 garlic cloves, minced

2 cups cannellini beans, drained and rinsed (roughly 1½ cans)

3 small Yellow or Red Bliss potatoes, cut into ½-inch cubes

3 cups vegetable broth

1 teaspoon fresh thyme leaves

Sea salt and pepper

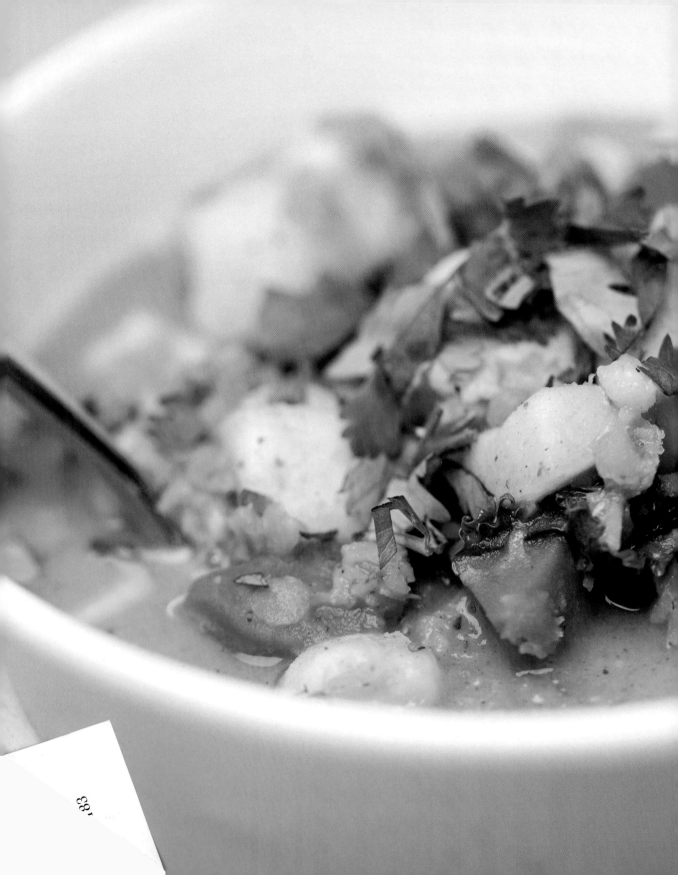

Red Lentil Curry Stew

This comforting stew is fiber and protein rich. Kale, cilantro, and curry seasoning are all great for helping the body purge toxins. Enjoy this on top of quinoa or brown rice.

1) Melt the oil in a large stockpot over medium heat. Add the onion and garlic and sauté until soft. Add the curry and cumin and stir to combine to release the flavors of the spices.

2) Add the carrots, cauliflower, and yam, and stir to incorporate the spices and vegetables. Add the lentils and broth. Turn the heat to high and bring to a boil. Once boiling, lower the heat to a simmer, cover, and let simmer for about 30 minutes or until the veggies are soft and the lentils are mushy.

3) Remove from the heat and add the coconut milk, kale, and cilantro. Season with salt and pepper.

4 Servings

1 tablespoon coconut oil

1 medium yellow onion, diced

3 garlic cloves, minced

2 tablespoons curry powder

1 teaspoon cumin

3 large carrots, cut into ¼-inch rounds

½ head cauliflower, cut into small florets

1 medium Japanese yam *or* garnet yam, peeled and cubed into ¼-inch pieces

1 cup red lentils

4 cups vegetable broth

1 cup canned coconut milk

2 cups chopped curly kale

1 handful cilantro, chopped

Sea salt and pepper

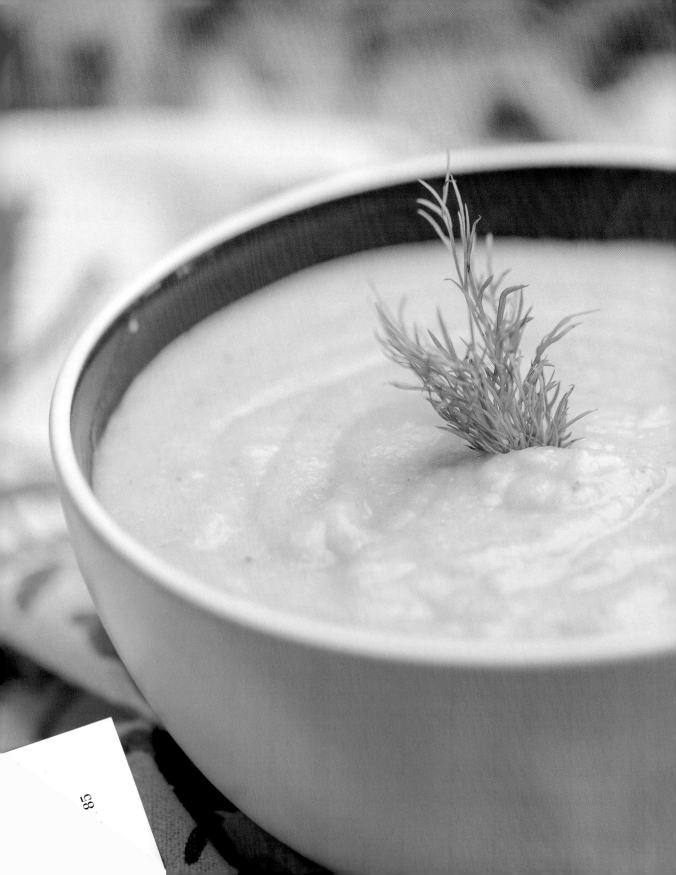

Creamy Cauliflower Soup

1) Melt the oil in a large stockpot over medium heat.

2) Add the garlic, leek, celery, and onion, and sauté until soft. Add the cauliflower, potatoes, and broth and stir. Turn the heat to high and bring to a boil.

3) Once boiling, lower the heat to a simmer, cover, and let simmer for about 30 minutes or until the veggies are soft.

4) Remove from the heat then add dill and stir to combine. Season with salt and pepper.

4 Servings

1 tablespoon coconut oil

2 garlic cloves, minced

½ small leek, white parts only, sliced thin

¼ cup diced celery

½ medium yellow onion, diced

1 small head cauliflower, cut into florets

4 Yellow Bliss potatoes, cubed

4 cups vegetable broth

¼ cup freshly chopped dill

Salt and pepper

Main Meals and Delightful Bowls

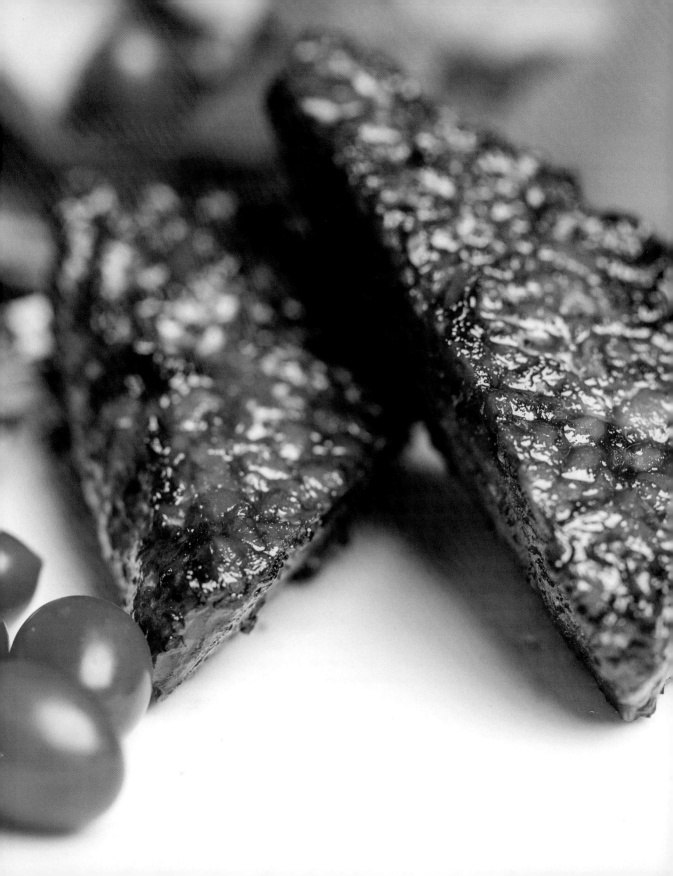

Maple-Glazed Baked Tempeh

This delicious tempeh dish is high in protein and a great substitute for any meat dish. It's sweet and tangy, and great to throw on top of a salad or some gluten-free grains.

1) Cut the tempeh into four triangles and place them in a baking dish. Blend the marinade ingredients in a blender and pour over the tempeh. Marinate for 30 minutes to 1 hour in the refrigerator.

2) Preheat the oven to 350 degrees F. Remove the tempeh from the refrigerator, cover the baking dish with foil, and bake for 15 minutes.

3) Remove the foil and bake for 5 more minutes. Be sure not to overbake, as it will dry out.

2 Servings

1 package (8 ounces) **tempeh**

Marinade:

3 tablespoons **low-sodium tamari**

3 tablespoons **maple syrup**

1 tablespoon **rice vinegar**

2 teaspoons **balsamic vinegar**

2 tablespoons **olive oil**

2 cloves **garlic**, peeled, crushed, and chopped

⅛ teaspoon **powdered chipotle**

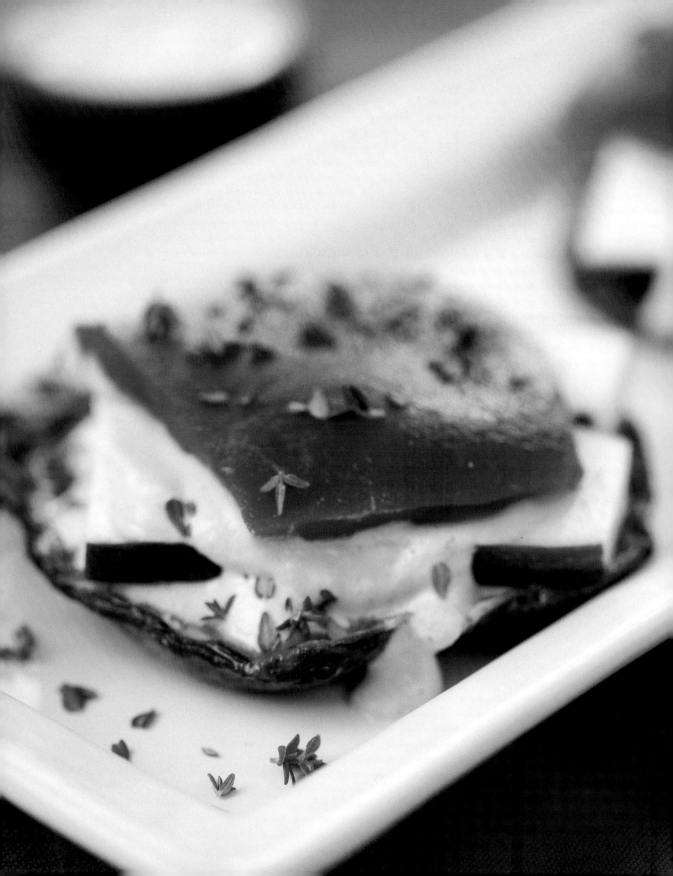

Portobello Stacker with Chipotle Cashew Cheese

This delicious entrée will make you feel as if you are eating a gourmet meal at a fancy restaurant. Even though it has simple ingredients, the health benefits are phenomenal.

1) Preheat the oven to 400 degrees F. Place the mushrooms in a baking dish cap side down with the zucchini slices. Cut the bell pepper into strips and set aside.

2) Whisk or blend together all the marinade ingredients in a large bowl and pour over the mushrooms and zucchini. Let this sit for 10 minutes.

3) Bake the mushrooms and zucchini in the oven for about 15 to 20 minutes or until soft and juicy. Remove from the oven.

To assemble the stackers, place one mushroom on a plate and spread a thin layer of the cashew cheese over the top. Add a few of the roasted bell pepper strips and a dollop of the Chipotle Cashew Cheese. Finish off by topping the stack with several zucchini strips. Season with salt and pepper, if desired.

2 Servings

2 large **portobello mushrooms**, stems removed

1 large **zucchini**, cut in half and sliced into ½-inch strips

1 roasted **red bell pepper**

Marinade:

3 tablespoons **extra virgin olive oil**

2 teaspoons **maple syrup**

1 tablespoon **Dijon mustard**

1 tablespoon **Bragg's Liquid Aminos**

1 tablespoon **apple cider vinegar**

¼ cup filtered **water**

2 **garlic cloves**, minced

2 tablespoons **balsamic vinegar**

1 teaspoon **dried oregano**

2 teaspoons freshly chopped **rosemary**

Chipotle Cashew Cheese (see recipe on p. 195)

Sea salt and **fresh cracked pepper**

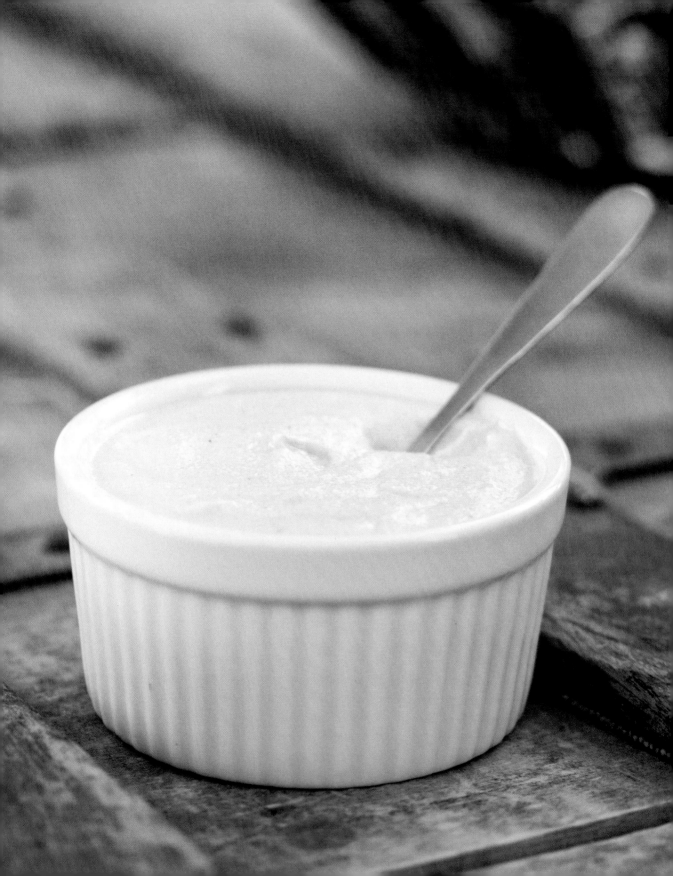

Chipotle Cashew Cheese

This vegan take on cheese sauce is delicious on just about everything. Cashews are high in magnesium and potassium, lending to your body's mineral balance.

1) Drain the water from the cashews and place all the ingredients in a blender with just enough water to barely cover. Blend until very smooth. Add more water if the mixture is too thick or if you're having trouble blending the ingredients. This sauce should be fairly thick.

6 to 8 Servings

1½ cups **cashews**, soaked in water for 1 hour

¼ cup **nutritional yeast flakes**

1 tablespoon **lemon juice**

½ teaspoon **chipotle chili powder**

½ teaspoon **garlic powder**

½ teaspoon **sea salt**

¼ teaspoon **smoked paprika** (optional)

Filtered **water**

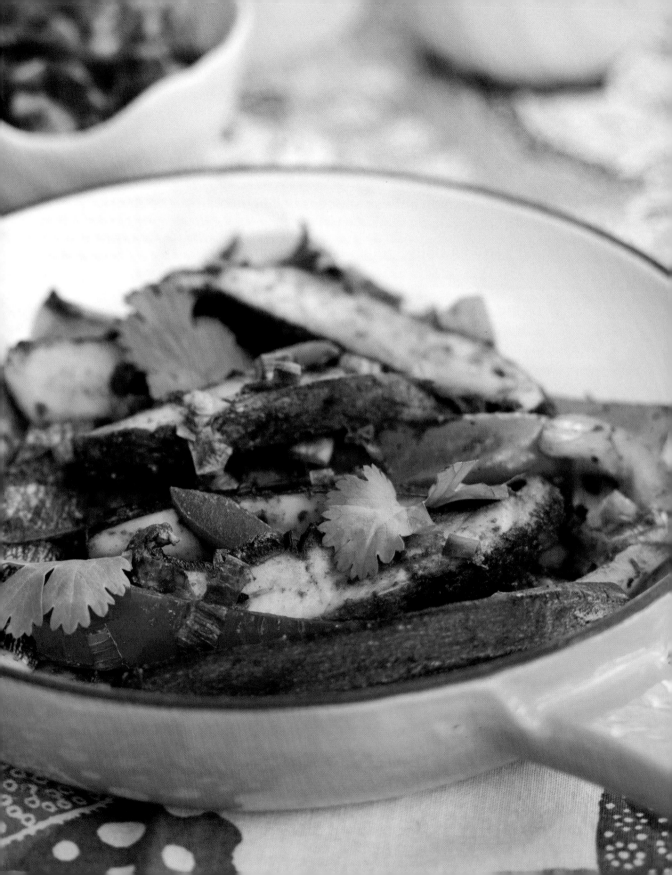

Veggie Fajita Wraps

Fajitas are a great way to get a lot of veggies together in one dish. These yummy wraps are healthy for you, loaded with fiber, and full of flavor.

1) Heat the oil in a large skillet over medium heat and sauté the onion and mushrooms. Cook for a few minutes until the onions are soft and the mushrooms have released their juices.

2) Add the bell peppers, zucchini, cumin, oregano, chili powder, and cilantro. Season with salt, if desired. Stir well to incorporate. Cover the skillet to let the veggies steam for about 5 to 7 minutes, stirring occasionally.

3) To assemble the fajitas, lay a collard leaf on a flat surface. Place a scoop of the fajita mixture on the bottom third of the leaf. Top with ¼ cup of the rice and two or three avocado slices. Roll up the leaf tightly while tucking in the sides.

2 Servings

1 tablespoon **extra virgin olive oil**

½ medium **yellow onion**, thinly sliced

1 large **portobello mushroom**, thinly sliced

½ **red bell pepper**, deseeded and thinly sliced

½ **green bell pepper**, deseeded and thinly sliced

½ medium **zucchini**, cut into ½-inch strips

1 teaspoon **cumin**

½ teaspoon **dried oregano**

2 teaspoons **chili powder**

Juice of 1 medium **lime**
   (about 1½ to 2 tablespoons)

2 tablespoons freshly **chopped cilantro**

Sea salt

½ cup cooked **brown rice**

Avocado slices

4 **collard green leaves**, de-stemmed

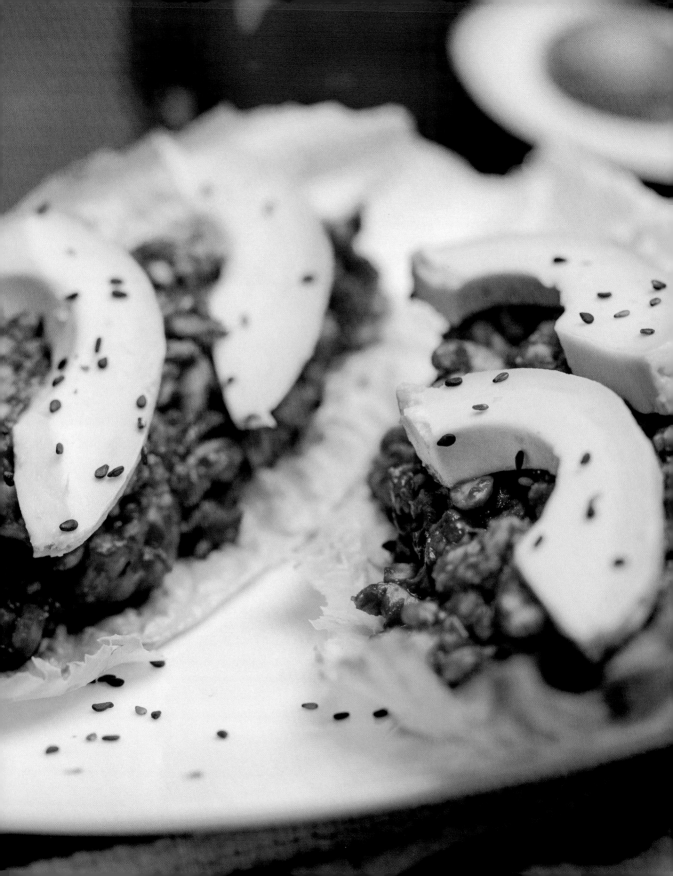

Sweet and Savory Tempeh Tacos

This fresh and zingy take on everyday tacos will have you hooked. The high-protein tempeh crumbles resemble the texture of ground meat. You won't even know you're not eating the real thing.

1) Heat 2 teaspoons of the oil in a large skillet over medium heat. Add the crumbled tempeh and sauté until lightly brown, stirring frequently.

2) In a small bowl, whisk together the remaining oil, Worcestershire sauce, tomato paste, sesame seeds, vinegar, and syrup. Pour the sauce over the tempeh and let the mixture cook for about 3 to 4 minutes or until the sauce is absorbed into the tempeh.

3) To assemble the tacos, place a spoonful of meat on a lettuce leaf and top with the avocado slices.

3 Servings (2 "tacos" each)

1 tablespoon plus 2 teaspoons **olive oil**

1 package *(8 ounces)* **tempeh,** crumbled

2 tablespoons **vegan Worcestershire sauce**

3 tablespoons **tomato paste**

2 tablespoons **sesame seeds**

2 tablespoons **apple cider vinegar**

2 teaspoons **maple syrup**

6 **Bibb** *or* **romaine lettuce** leaves

Avocado slices

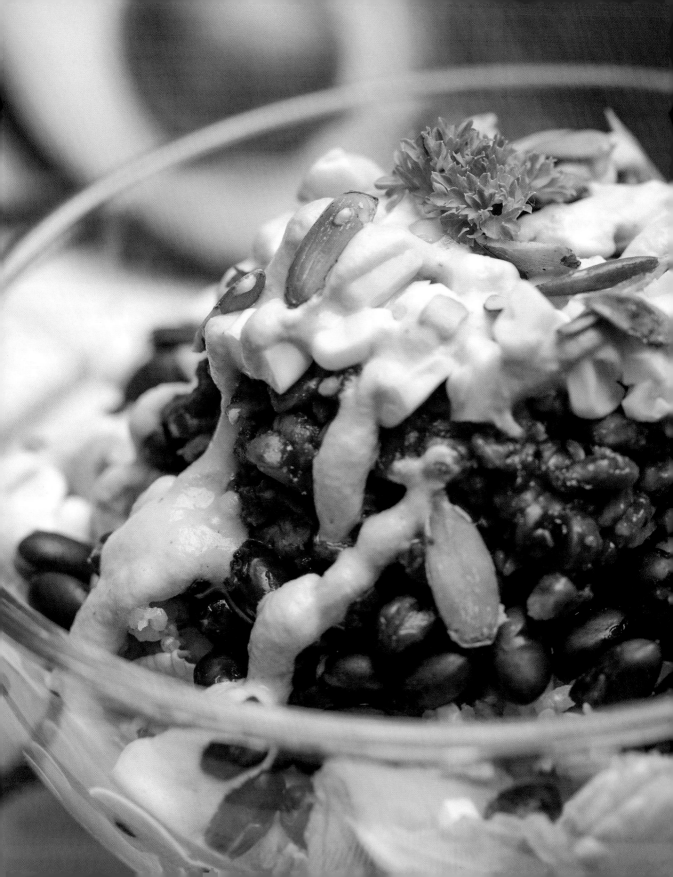

Taco Salad Bowl with Smoky Chipotle Dressing

This bowl is one of my favorites, as it's filling, full of flavor, and easy to throw together. Add a couple of avocado slices on top for extra added healthy fats.

1) Put the salad ingredients in a bowl. Blend the dressing ingredients together in a blender until smooth and creamy. This dressing will be thick. If you like a thinner dressing, add 1 to 2 tablespoons of water and reblend. Pour the dressing over the salad.

1 Serving

Salad:

2 cups chopped **romaine lettuce**

1 scoop **Sweet and Savory taco "meat"**

½ cup **black beans**

2 tablespoons **toasted pumpkin seeds**

½ cup fresh, raw **corn, off the cob**

¼ cup cooked **brown rice**

Smoky Chipotle Dressing:

¼ cup tahini

2 tablespoons **extra virgin olive oil**

3 tablespoons **apple cider vinegar**

2 tablespoons **maple syrup**

2 tablespoons filtered **water**

Juice of 1 medium **lemon** (*about 3 tablespoons*)

⅛ teaspoon **chipotle chili powder**

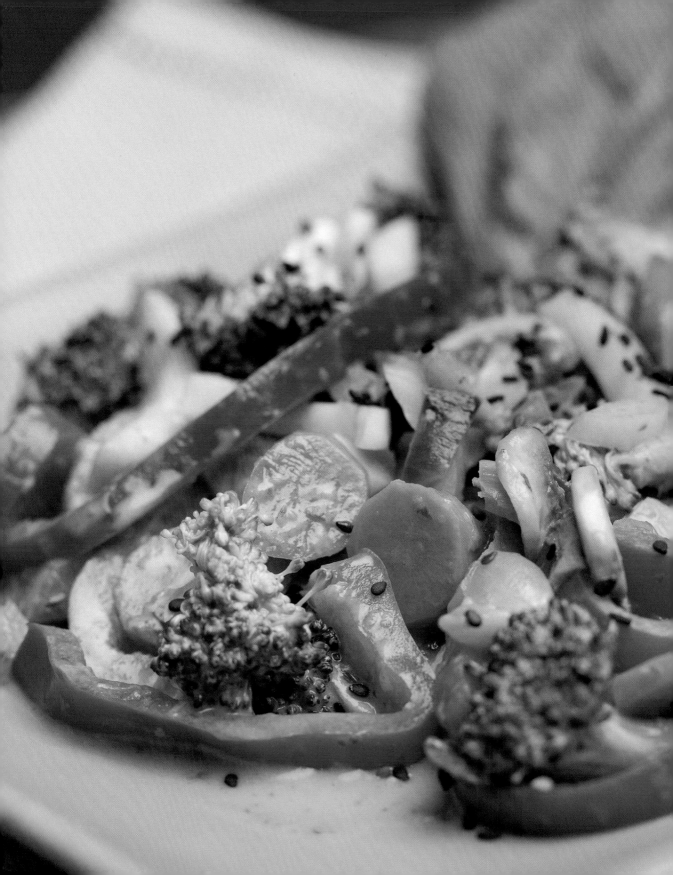

Coconut Basil Stir-Fry

Creamy coconut basil sauce is perfect on top of high-antioxidant fresh veggies. Stir-fries are so simple to make. You can use any combination of veggies you like. Get creative! It's a win/win, no matter what.

1) Put the coconut sauce ingredients in a blender and blend to combine. Set aside.

2) To prepare the stir-fry, heat the oil in a large wok or a sauté pan over medium-high heat. Sauté the garlic and onion until translucent. Add the ginger and sauté for another minute. Add the carrots, bell pepper, and mushrooms. Cook for another 3 minutes. Add the broccoli and bok choy, and stir to combine.

3) Pour the coconut sauce over the veggies. Cover the pan with a lid, reduce the heat to medium, and let the veggies steam in the sauce for a few minutes until the sauce begins to thicken. Stir occasionally. Do not overcook the vegetables or let them get soggy. Serve over quinoa.

4 Servings

Coconut Sauce:

1 cup chopped fresh **basil leaves**

1 cup regular **coconut milk**

2 tablespoons **Bragg's Liquid Aminos**

1 tablespoon fresh **lime juice**

2 tablespoons **rice vinegar**

1 teaspoon **arrowroot powder**

1 tablespoon **maple syrup**

Stir-Fry:

1 tablespoon **coconut oil**

2 cloves **garlic**, minced

¼ cup diced **red onion**

1 teaspoon grated **fresh ginger**

4 medium **carrots**, halved and cut into ¼-inch diagonal slices

1 **red bell pepper**, deseeded and cut into strips

1 cup thinly sliced **mushrooms**

1 cup **broccoli florets**

1 cup thinly sliced **bok choy** or **cabbage**

2 cups cooked **quinoa**

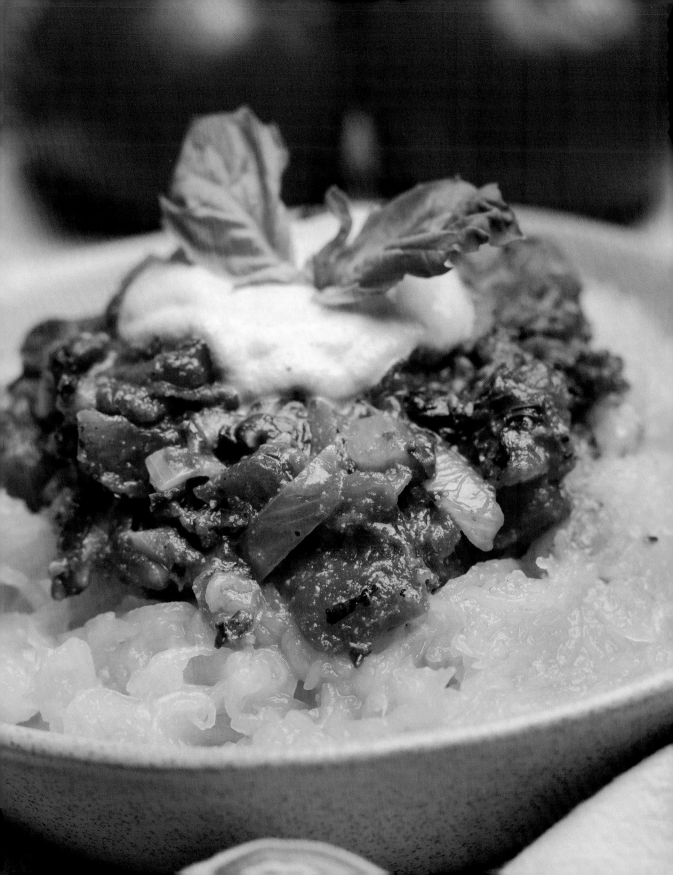

Spaghetti Squash Italiano

A perfect replacement for highly processed pasta, this dish will leave you feeling satisfied and happy. You may never eat pasta again!

1) Preheat the oven to 375 degrees F. Place the squash in a large baking dish, cut side down. Add about ½ inch of water to the dish. Bake for about 40 minutes or until the squash is fork-tender. Remove it from the oven and let it cool slightly. Using a spoon, gently scrape out the seeds and discard. Using a fork, scrape out the spaghetti-like strands and discard the skins. Set the squash aside.

2) Heat the oil in a skillet and sauté the garlic and onion with the red pepper flakes until the onions are soft and slightly caramelized.

3) Add the mushrooms, spinach, oregano, basil, and vinegar. Stir to combine and cook for about 5 minutes or until the mushrooms cook down and the spinach wilts.

4) Add the tomatoes, nutritional yeast, salt, and pepper, and cook for about 7 more minutes to let the tomatoes simmer and meld with the flavors. Serve on top of the warm squash with a dollop of Chipotle Cashew Cheese.

2 to 3 Servings

1 small **spaghetti squash**, cut in half lengthwise

1 tablespoon **extra virgin olive oil**

2 **garlic cloves**, minced

½ cup finely diced **red onion**

¼ teaspoon crushed **red pepper flakes**

4 small **mushrooms**, roughly chopped

1 cup finely chopped **fresh spinach**

1 teaspoon **dried oregano**

1 teaspoon **dried basil**

2 teaspoons **red wine vinegar**

1 can *(15 ounces)* **fire-roasted diced tomatoes**

2 tablespoons **nutritional yeast**

½ teaspoon **sea salt**

Freshly **ground pepper**

Chipotle Cashew Cheese *(see recipe on p. 195)*

Spaghetti Squash Surprise Bowl

A perfectly satisfying meal with lots of texture and flavor. Go ahead and use any greens you have on hand and be generous with the mineral-rich Chipotle Cashew Cheese.

1) Put all the ingredients except the Chipotle Cashew Cheese in a bowl. Drizzle the Chipotle Cashew Cheese over the top.

1 Serving

1 cup leftover **Spaghetti Squash Italiano** *(see recipe on p. 205)*

¼ cup leftover **Herbed Brown Rice and Lentil Salad** *(see recipe on p. 151)*

½ cup chopped **curly kale**

Chipotle Cashew Cheese *(see recipe on p. 195)*

Indian Spiced Baked Yam with Coconut Oil

Yams are a great way to tame your sweet tooth while adding an awesome dose of muscle-fueling complex carbohydrates to your diet. The coconut oil will aid in burning fat—a double bonus!

1) Preheat the oven to 400 degrees F. Clean the yam and poke holes in it with a fork. Place it on a baking sheet and bake it for 30 to 40 minutes or until soft.

2) Remove it from the oven and place it in a bowl. Slit the yam open down the middle and add the oil, garam masala, and sea salt.

3) Use a fork to mush the flavors into the flesh of the yam.

1 Serving

1 medium **garnet yam**

2 teaspoons **coconut oil**

¼ teaspoon **garam masala**

Sea salt

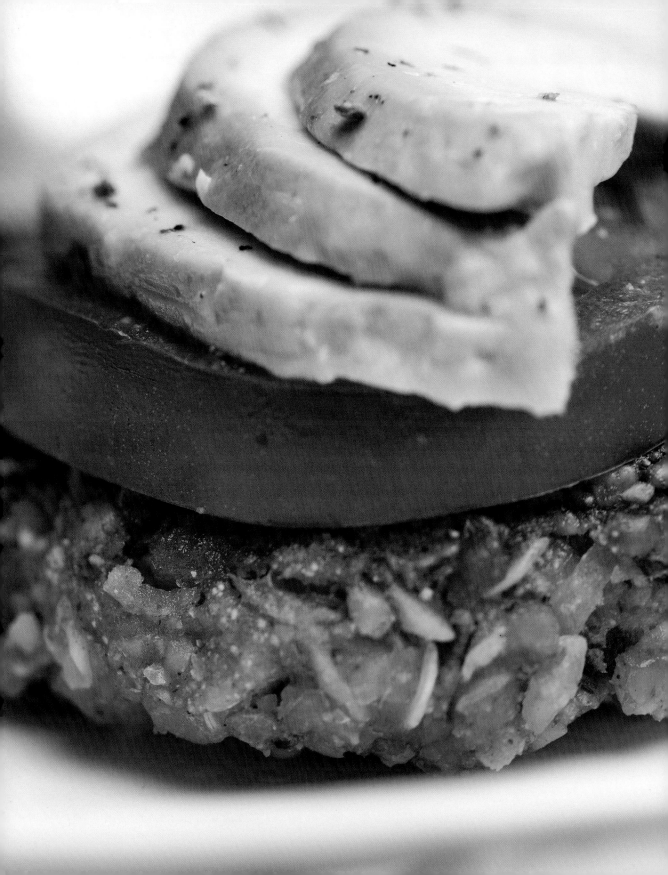

Curried Red Lentil Walnut Burger

This delicious lentil walnut burger contains fiber, healthy fats, and protein. The spices in the curry seasoning are warming to the system and help cleanse your digestive tract as well.

1) Combine the lentils and broth in a saucepan and bring to a boil. Reduce the heat and simmer for about 20 minutes or until the lentils are soft. Strain the lentils to remove excess water and set aside to cool.

2) Heat 2 teaspoons of the coconut oil in a sauté pan and sauté the onions, peppers, and garlic until soft. Add the curry powder and stir to combine well. Remove from the heat and set aside.

3) Put the lentils, walnuts, and rice in the bowl of a food processor and process until textured but not gooey. Transfer to a bowl and add the onion, pepper, garlic, and bread crumbs or oat flour, and salt. Stir well to combine.

4) Heat the remaining oil in a skillet. Form six patties and brown them over medium heat. If the mixture is too sticky, wet your hands. If it's too dry, add 1 tablespoon of water at a time until it's the desired consistency.

5) Wrap the mixture in lettuce leaves or serve on a bed of spinach/kale and top with slices of onion, avocado, and tomato.

6 Servings

½ cup **red lentils**

1 cup **vegetable broth**

1 tablespoon **coconut oil**

1 small **red onion**, diced

1 **red bell pepper**, diced

2 **cloves garlic**, minced

2 teaspoons **curry powder**

½ cup **raw walnuts**

½ cup cooked **brown rice**

¼ cup **gluten-free bread crumbs** *or* **oat flour**

1 teaspoon **sea salt**

Optional: lettuce leaves or kale, slice of onion, tomato, or avocado

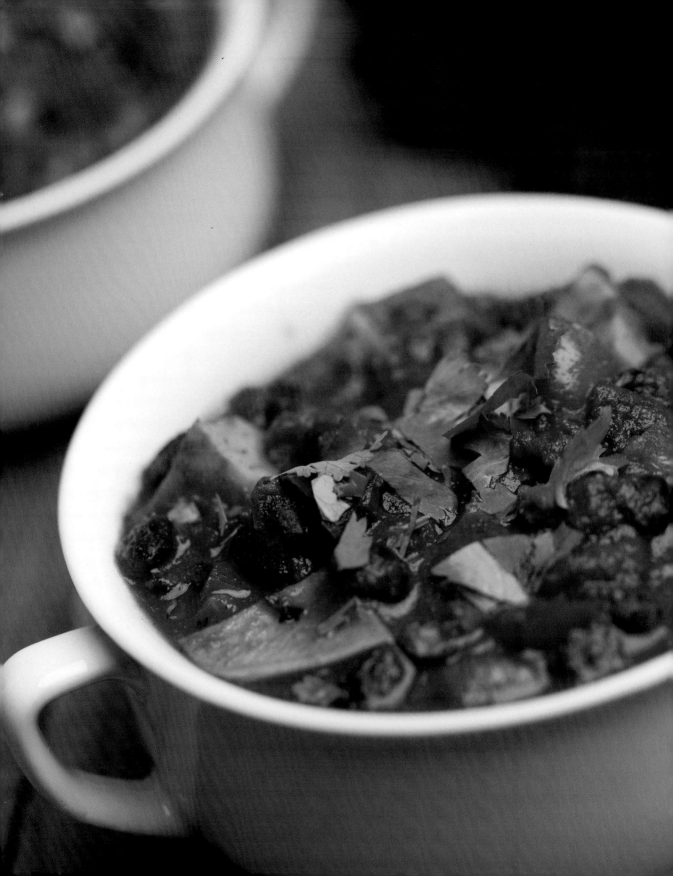

Karma Black Bean Chili

This chili has a sweet and healthy twist: garnet yams. Fiber-rich and loaded with complex carbs, it will satisfy you and help your body burn fat.

1) Heat the oil in a large pot over medium heat and sauté the garlic, onion, bell pepper, and sea salt until soft (about 4 to 5 minutes).

2) Add the cumin and chili powder and stir to combine. Cook for another minute.

3) Add the yam, tomatoes, beans, lime juice, and water. Stir well to combine. Bring to a simmer, cover, and cook for about 20 minutes, or until potatoes are soft. Top with cilantro, if desired, when serving.

4 Servings

1 tablespoon **coconut oil**

2 **garlic cloves**, minced

½ medium **red onion**, diced

½ **red bell pepper**, deseeded and diced

1 teaspoon **sea salt**

2 teaspoons **cumin**

1 tablespoon **chili powder**

1 large **garnet yam**, peeled and cut into ½-inch cubes

1 can *(28 ounces)* **fire-roasted crushed tomatoes**

2 cans *(15 ounces each)* **black beans**, drained and rinsed

Juice of 1 medium **lime** *(about 1½ to 2 tablespoons)*

¼ cup **water**

¼ cup chopped **cilantro** *(optional)*

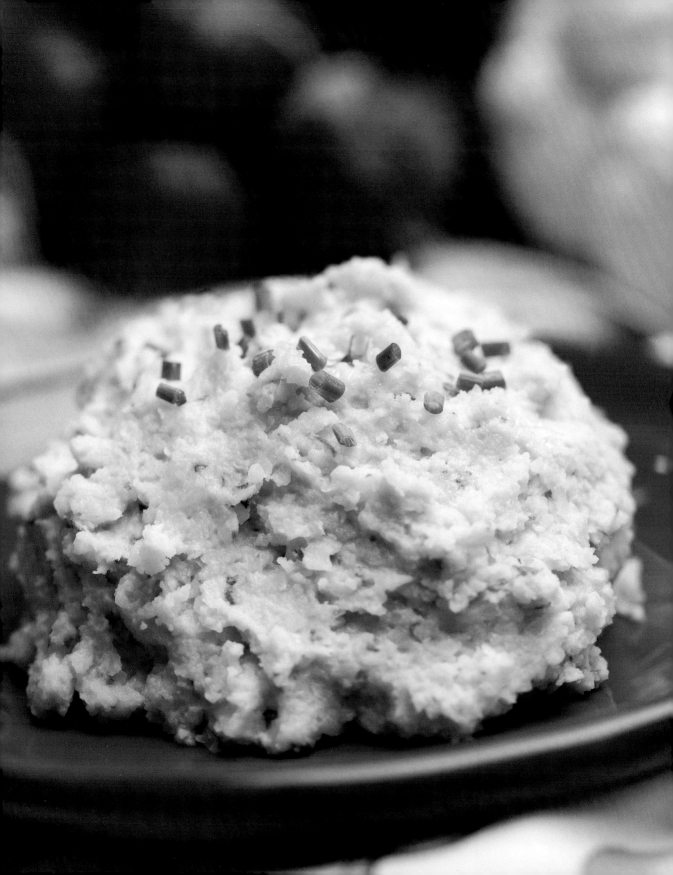

Roasted Root Veggies

Kidney-tonifying root veggies roasted in the oven taste just like candy in my book. Eating these complex carbohydrate jewels will satisfy your sweet tooth and give you energy to burn.

1) Preheat the oven to 400 degrees F. Put the veggies in a bowl and drizzle with enough olive oil to coat them. Season with salt and the herbs of your choice. Bake in the oven for about 20 to 30 minutes or until the veggies are soft, slightly brown, and caramelized.

2 Servings

½ large **garnet yam**, peeled and cubed

1 large **parsnip**, peeled and cubed

2 large **carrots**, cut into ½-inch chunks

1 large **red** or **yellow beet**, peeled and cubed

3 small **red potatoes**, cubed

½ large **yellow onion**, cut in chunks

Olive oil

Sea salt

Dried herbs of your choice
(I like a combination of marjoram, basil, and thyme)

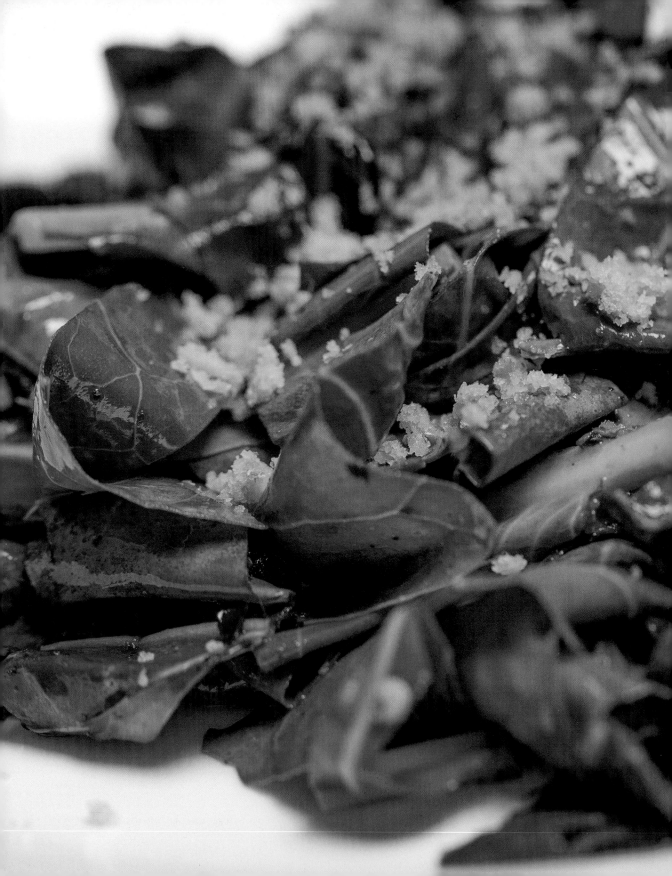

Spicy Home-Style Collards

In the South, collard greens are usually cooked in lard and topped with bacon. They are one of the highest nutrient leafy greens you can eat. This healthy and delicious version will turn you into a collard convert.

1) Melt the oil in a skillet over medium heat. Sauté the garlic and onions until soft. Add the red pepper flakes and paprika, and stir to combine. Add the collard greens and apple cider vinegar and cook until slightly wilted but still bright green. Add sea salt to taste. Top with the "Cheese" Sprinkles.

3 Servings

1 tablespoon **coconut oil**

2 **garlic cloves**, minced

⅓ cup diced **red onion**

Pinch of **red pepper flakes**

¼ teaspoon **smoked paprika**

1 bunch of **collard greens**, stems removed and chopped

1 tablespoon **apple cider vinegar**

Sea salt

"Cheese" Sprinkles *(see recipe on p. 155)*

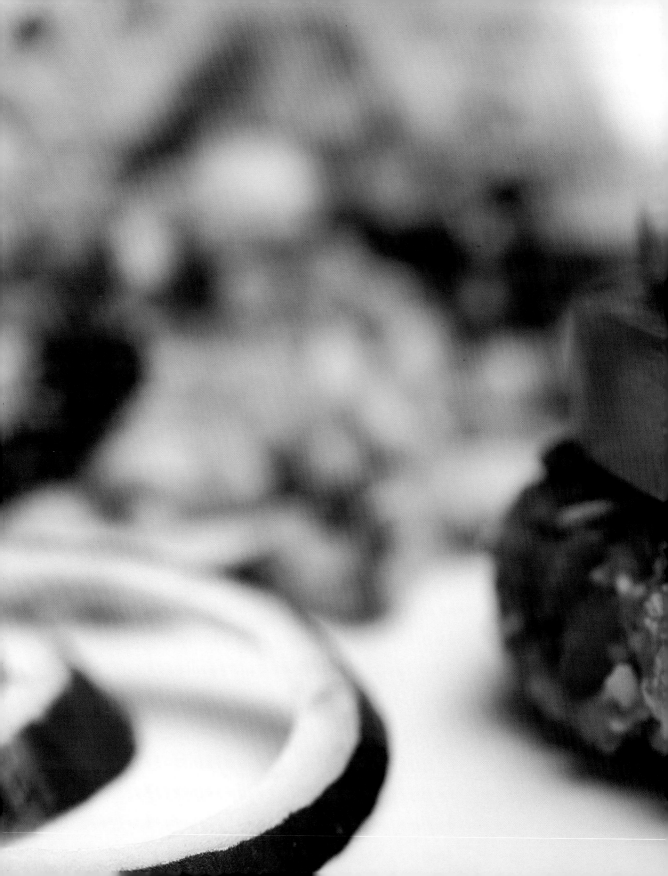

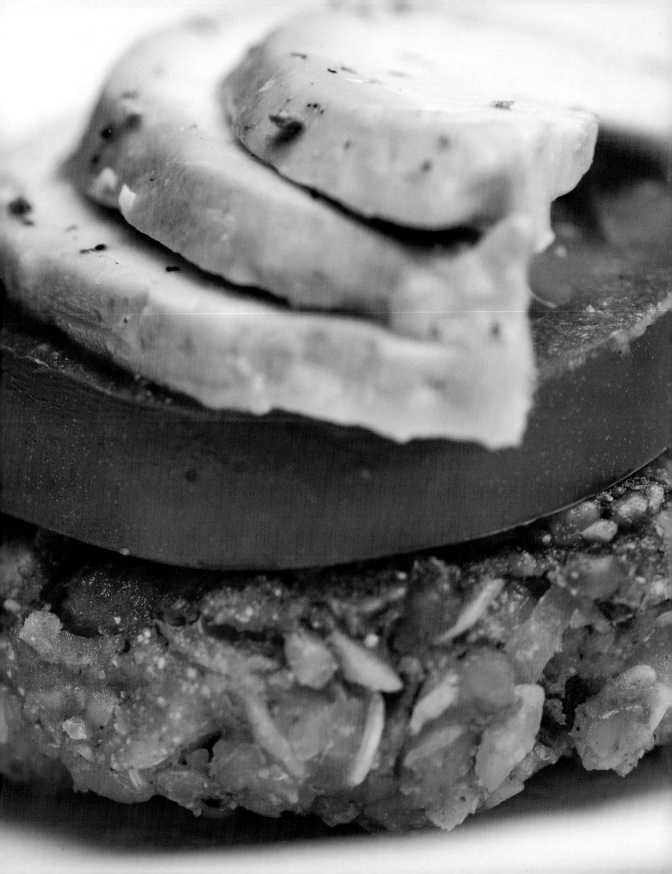

Delectable Dips for Snacking

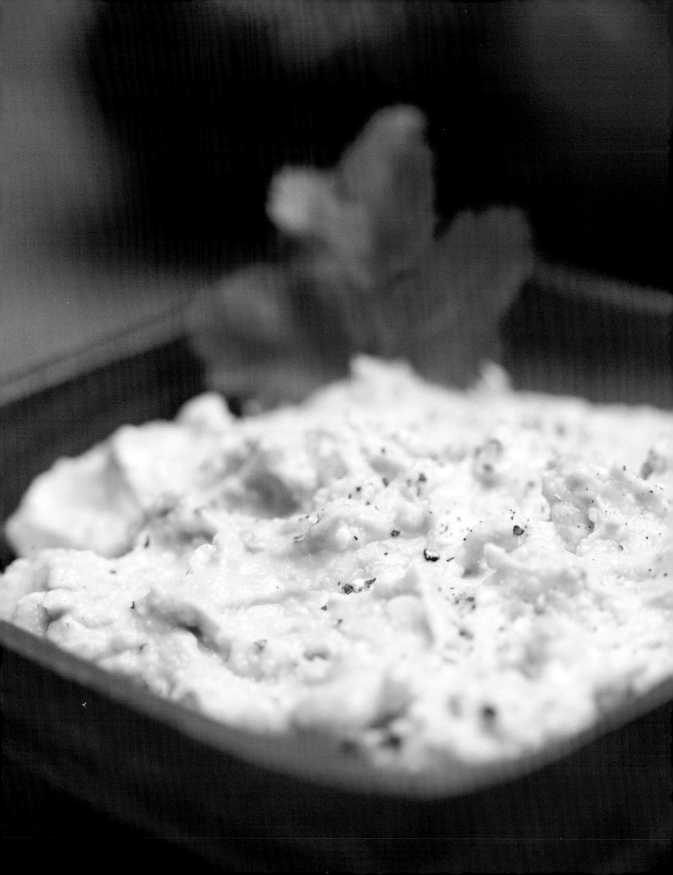

Sofia's Glowing Guac

My sweet friend Sofia, who is only nine, came up with this awesome guacamole recipe, which is packed full of flavor and nutrients. Avocados help your skin glow from the inside out.

1) Put the avocados in a bowl and mash them until smooth. Add the remaining ingredients and stir well to combine.

4 to 6 Servings

2 ripe **avocados**, pits removed

1 **garlic** clove, minced small

2 tablespoons finely **minced onion**

3 dashes **Tabasco** or ¼ teaspoon **minced jalapeño**

2 teaspoons **lemon juice**

¼ teaspoon **salt**

Freshly **ground pepper**

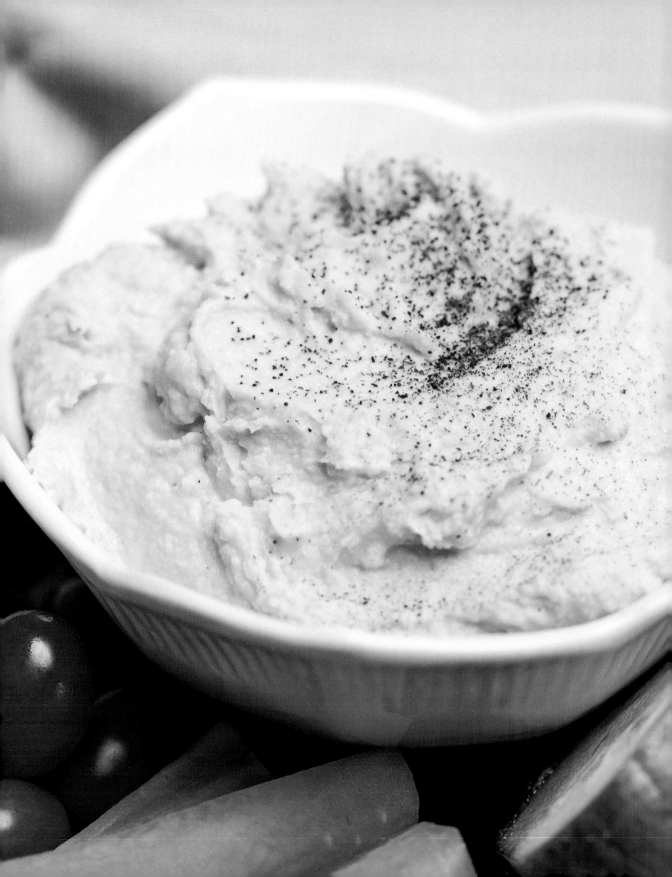

Garlicky Hummus

Hummus is an awesome snack with fresh veggies, because it provides a good dose of protein, complex carbs, and fiber.

1) Put all the ingredients except the oil into a food processor bowl fitted with an S-curve blade and puree, scraping down the bowl as needed. With the motor running, drizzle the oil through the feed tube until the hummus is creamy smooth.

4 to 6 Servings

1 can *(15 ounces)* **chickpeas**, drained and rinsed

1 tablespoon **tahini**

2 **cloves garlic**

Juice of 1 **medium lemon** *(about 3 tablespoons)*

1 teaspoon **cumin**

½ teaspoon **sea salt**

3 tablespoons **olive oil**

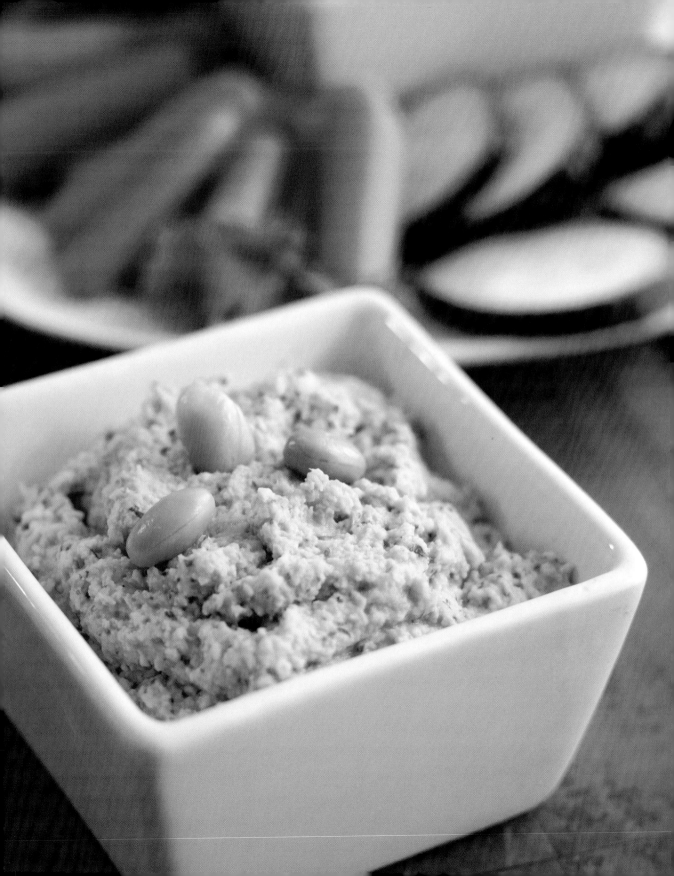

Kickin' Edamame Dip

Edamame, also known as soybean, is high in fiber and protein. It's easily found in your grocer's freezer, but make sure you buy preshelled edamame for ease. I also recommend buying organic, as oftentimes nonorganic contains genetically modified organisms (GMOs).

1) Put all of the ingredients into a food processor except for the olive oil and lime juice. Puree until combined.

2) Add the olive oil and lime juice and puree more, scraping the sides of the processor bowl frequently. If you like a smoother consistency, add purified water 1 tablespoon at a time while the processor is running, until the desired texture is achieved.

About 2 Cups

1 package (*16 ounces*) **frozen and shelled edamame**, cooked according to instructions

4 large **garlic cloves**, chopped

1¼ teaspoons **sea salt**

½ teaspoon ground **coriander**

1 teaspoon ground **cumin**

¼ teaspoon **cayenne**

¼ cup fresh **cilantro**

4–6 tablespoons **extra virgin olive oil**

¼ cup freshly squeezed **lime juice**

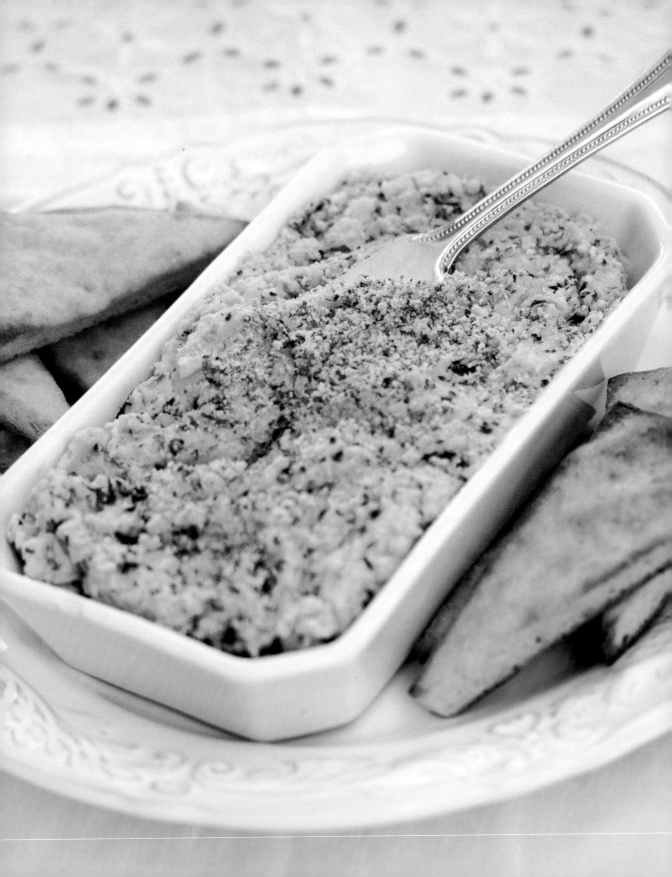

Creamy Spinach Artichoke Dip

High-fiber white beans, paired with naturally detoxifying artichokes, make this a healthy take on spinach artichoke dip—a perfect cleanse snack for your body.

1) Preheat the oven to 400 degrees F. Drain the cashews. In a food processor or blender, blend the cashews and beans with the water, lemon juice, Vegenaise, and nutritional yeast until creamy. If mixture is too thick, add water 1 tablespoon at a time until thick and creamy. Scrape into a bowl and set aside.

2) Heat the olive oil in a skillet over medium heat and sauté the onion and garlic until soft. Add the artichokes and sauté until lightly browned. Add the spinach and let it wilt down, about 2 to 3 minutes.

3) Pour into a large bowl and add the cashew and bean mixture, salt, and red pepper flakes (to taste). Stir to combine well.

4) Pour into a lightly oiled casserole dish and top with bread crumbs. Cover with foil and bake for about 15 minutes. Remove foil and bake 10 minutes more until a little browned.

About 2 Cups

½ cup **cashews**, soaked for 20 minutes

1 15-ounce can **cannellini** (*white*) beans, drained and rinsed

½ cup **water**

2 tablespoons **lemon juice**

¼ cup **grapeseed Vegenaise**

3 tablespoons **nutritional yeast**

1 tablespoon **extra virgin olive oil**

1 medium **yellow onion**, diced

4 **garlic cloves**, minced

1½ cups thawed and chopped frozen **artichoke hearts** (*or substitute 1½ cups jarred artichoke hearts*)

3 cups chopped fresh **spinach** (*chopped small*)

1 teaspoon **sea salt**

Dash **red pepper flakes**

¼ cup **gluten-free bread crumbs**

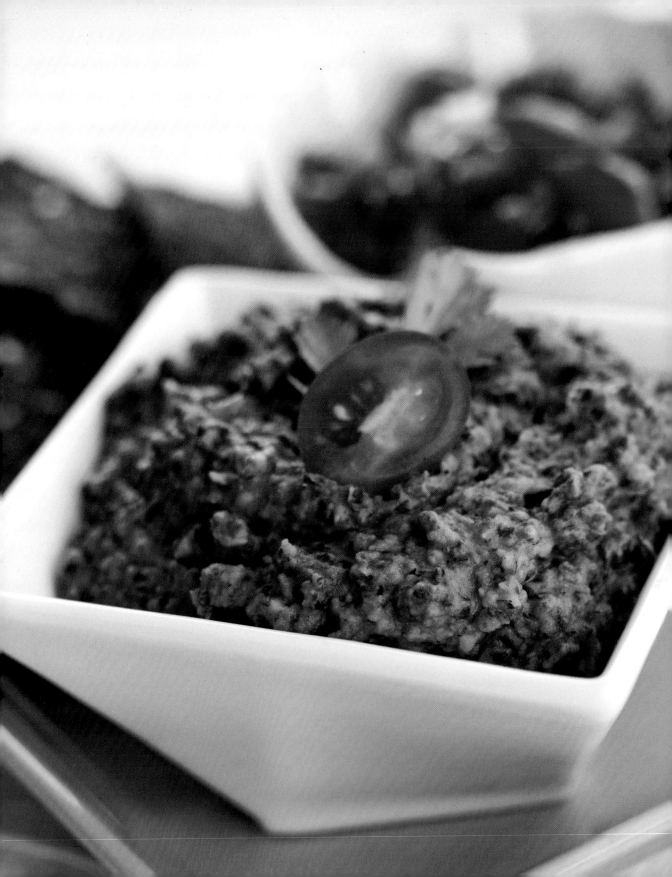

Arriba Black Bean Dip

This dip is smoky, spicy, and just plain great! Serve it with some baked blue corn chips or cut-up veggies. It will transport you right to the sandy beaches of Mexico!

1) Heat 1 tablespoon of the olive oil in a skillet over medium heat and sauté the jalapeño, red bell pepper, onion, and garlic until soft. Add the cumin and chili powder and stir while cooking to incorporate. Remove from heat when all of the ingredients are soft and somewhat caramelized.

2) In a food processor, place the pepper mixture, black beans, apple cider vinegar, honey, and salt. Puree all of the ingredients while pouring the remaining 2 tablespoons of olive oil into the processor while running. Make sure you remove the lid and scrape the sides and puree again. Serve warm or chilled.

About 3 Cups

3 tablespoons **olive oil**

½ **jalapeño pepper**, deseeded and minced

1 **red bell pepper**, deseeded and diced

1 small **red onion**, finely diced

1 **garlic** clove, minced

1 teaspoon **cumin**

¼ teaspoon **chipotle chili powder**

1½ cups **canned black beans**, rinsed

1 tablespoon **apple cider vinegar**

2 teaspoons **honey** or **maple syrup**

½ teaspoon **sea salt**

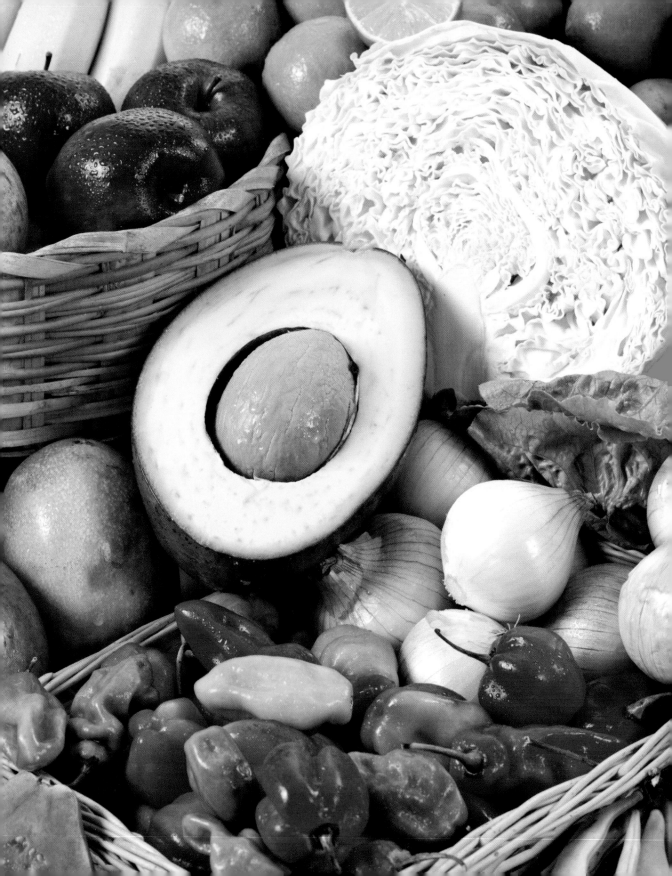

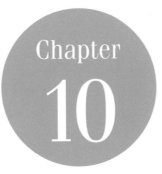

Chapter 10

Post-Clean in 14 Transition Guidelines

Yahoo!!! You have done it. You have completed the Clean in 14 Program. I want you to take a moment and acknowledge yourself and the commitment you made to your health and well-being! Pat yourself on the back. Brag out loud to your friends. Do a happy dance. Seriously. Do whatever it is you need to do to celebrate your courage, commitment, and perseverance. You truly are amazing!

For these last 14 days, you have been putting super, squeaky-clean food into your body. If you followed along like a good student, then you are probably noticing some pretty significant changes in your body, mood, weight, and more. Maybe these changes are subtle, and if so, that's okay too. Whatever they are, they are meant to be celebrated and not taken lightly. A lot of change happens under the surface that you may not be seeing right now. Remember that this is only the beginning. Your body will only continue to change more and more as you stay on this path. Maybe you didn't drop as much weight as you would've liked or your energy is still not where you want it to be. That's okay, because as you continue on with this way of living, your body will continue to change, transform, and heal. Remember, it took years of abuse to get your body in the sickly, overweight state it was in when you started, so it will take time to undo it all and get your body back to its natural, healthy state.

These guidelines are here to help you as you transition, and encourage you so that you can continue this way of eating and make it your lifestyle. I want this for you, because I want you to be as healthy, vital, happy, and energetic as you deserve to be. And this doesn't mean you have to be vegan or never eat sugar again, but what it does mean is that you have taken serious steps in starting to heal your body, so there's no sense in throwing it all away when it's only just beginning and you may not even know what is possible for you!

I cannot stress enough how important preventative action is to your life and your health. This way of eating is not only preventative, but it will support your body, mind, and spirit in ways you didn't think were possible. It is a lifelong journey and one that has only just begun! I am so excited for all the doors that will continue to open for you as you continue forward.

How to Transition

Remember, it can be easy to slip back into your old habits, so make sure to keep yourself in check. Do your best to not give in to those unhealthy habits of the past that you have worked so hard to overcome these past few weeks. It can be a slippery slope once you start.

When transitioning out of the 14-day cleanse, it's best to do it slowly. I wouldn't encourage you to run out and add everything back into your diet that you cut out, because you could get very ill if you did that. Your body is a clean running machine right now, and it's going to be very sensitive to toxic foods.

This is a lifestyle, and you want to stay as close to the plan as possible. I am not saying that you need to be a vegan, or totally gluten free, but this way of eating has been proven to reverse diabetes, heart disease, and other diseases that the usual American diet cannot, as well as support longevity, vitality, and happiness.

Continue eating the way you have been and add back one food that you desire per week or every couple of days (e.g., fish, eggs, dairy, etc.). Do not do it all at once. You do not want to overload your clean, balanced body. My suggestion is that if you want to add animal products back into your diet, you buy only the highest-quality eggs, beef, fish, and so on, and that you only eat them two to four times per week maximum. This will ensure that your body stays clean and continues to work at its optimum level.

You may want to start dipping your fingers into certain foods or drinks you haven't been able to ingest for these last couple of weeks. What you may find is that (1) your body can no longer tolerate such food or drink and (2) you may not even like how some foods and drinks taste anymore. Your body will tell you pretty quickly if it likes them or not. *Pay attention* to that! If your body responds negatively to something, you have your answer as to whether it likes a certain food or not. Remember, our bodies may have a lot of sensitivities to foods that we didn't even know about, so when you add them back in and your body responds with bloating, gas, indigestion, headache, and so on, it may mean that your body does not like that food and that that food will not serve it in being the healthiest you can be.

I am not saying that you need to be a vegan, or totally gluten free, but this way of eating has been proven to reverse diabetes, heart disease, and other diseases that the usual American diet cannot, as well as support longevity, vitality, and happiness.

Hopefully, the longer you continue to eat clean, the more immune you will become to the world of unhealthy food around you. Soon enough, if you stay committed, you won't even notice the jar of candy on your coworker's desk or the box of doughnuts in the break room. This will take time, but it can definitely happen. It's best to have your list of nonnegotiables, which are foods you will not eat no matter what. Mine are white sugar, baked goods (unless they are Karma Chow, of course), and meat and dairy products. No matter what the occasion, I will not put these foods into my body, because I know exactly what the outcome will be. Remember in the beginning of the book when I talked about consequences and the 1 to 10 scale? This is a good way to continue forward on the path. Constantly revisit that scale and your nonnegotiable list. You will get clearer about what the nonnegotiables are as you move forward and your body starts to respond to what you put into it after completing this program.

Listen to the signs your body gives you and then make a decision moving forward about what works and what doesn't. Remember: it takes Patience, Persistence, and Commitment!

What to Stay Away From

There are certain foods and beverages that just do not serve us in maintaining a healthy body and vibrant life. These foods are best completely avoided or indulged in lightly (one or two times per month). Of course, always use your own discernment in any situation.

- **Coffee** is highly disruptive to our nervous system, as well as acidic in the body. It negatively affects our blood sugar balance and releases stress hormones into our system. *Healthier options:* green tea, Dandy Blend, Teeccino, and herbal teas.

- **Alcohol** is a depressant, and over time it can deplete serotonin (the feel-good chemical) in our body. Best to drink alcohol minimally, like one time per month or not at all. Yes, you can still go out and be social. This does not mean your social life is over; you are just making a healthier choice. *Healthier options:* wine spritzers or sparkling mineral water with cranberry juice and lime.

- **Soda** is *poison*, plain and simple—no explanation needed. *Healthier options:* water and herbal tea.

- **Artificial sweeteners** are *poison*! Do yourself a favor and stay away from these (including gum and mints). *Healthier options:* alternative, low-glycemic sweeteners listed on the "What to Enjoy" list (see Chapter 5), peppermint oil on your tongue, a sprig of parsley or fresh mint. If you must chew gum or eat mints, buy xylitol gum only (XyliChew is a good brand).

- **White sugar** will erode your body from the inside out. It feeds cancer cells and depresses the immune system for up to six hours after ingesting it. You now know what it's like to live without it—stick to it! There are plenty of healthier options out there. Always make the healthier choice! *Healthier options:* low-glycemic sweeteners (see the "What to Enjoy" list in Chapter 5) or any dessert from *The Karma Chow Ultimate Cookbook* or other gluten-free, low-glycemic options.

- **Processed foods:** To me, these foods are dead food or "frankenfood," but there are some nutrients in whole-grain products. Best to keep processed food to a bare minimum—shoot for the 95/5 or 90/10 rule! *Healthier options:* sprouted whole-grain and gluten-free breads, flours, raw crackers, and pastas.

Stay the Course: Continuing Practices

I cannot stress how important it is to stay on course with your new lifestyle and to continue to ingrain these new, healthier habits you have built. If you start to let them go, you will find yourself right back where you started. Make these activities part of your everyday life.

Batch Cooking and Planning

I encourage you to continue planning your meals each week and batch cooking. Eventually this will become easier for you, and sort of second nature. This is really the *only* way to ensure you will have healthy food available to you at all times! Sit down on Saturday morning and choose the meals you want for the week. Make your grocery list, hit the store, and come on home and cook it up. It feels so good to have deliciously prepared food waiting in your fridge for you when you come home from a long day at work!

Meditations

Continuing to use the guided meditations or your own source of meditation after these 14 days will not only help to solidify the new habits you have created but will help you manage the daily stressors in your life as well. Meditation has many positive benefits, and I encourage you to continue with this practice as much as possible. Make it part of your daily agenda. It's a great way to ground yourself and start or finish your day.

Journaling

During these 14 days you may have noticed some habits that have not necessarily served you. Whether you are an emotional eater, overeater, comfort seeker, or junk food junkie, these are habits that you most likely picked up as a child that can be hard to break. Continuing to journal is a great way to become aware of these patterns so that you can shift them and work with them. Flow and Go Writing is a very useful tool in helping to release any emotions you may have stored up or that you feel you cannot process. Remember to make sure that after you write it down, you rip it up or burn it to release the energy of it. I practice this type of writing almost daily, and it has changed my life in so many positive ways.

Impeccable Self-Care

Continue to do things that nurture your soul. Out of any of these practices, this is the *most* important. No matter how well you eat, if you do not take care of yourself on the mental, emotional, and spiritual levels, it will be much harder to stick to this new lifestyle! Schedule in your self-care weekly or daily if you can. This will ensure that you are taking care of yourself on every level and filling your soul so that you can be a better parent, friend, spouse, partner, and human being.

The Balance Practice

This is a great tool to work from to see where you need to find balance in your life. I would rewrite your list (see Day 9: Balance in Chapter 8) once a month to see which areas need your focus. Put your attention on the areas that need it. What can you do to shift these areas? What action steps can you take to bring more balance into those parts of your life? Make a commitment to yourself to work on this. Schedule it into your life!

Self-Appreciation

Along with impeccable self-care, the practice of self-appreciation (see Day 12: Self-Appreciation in Chapter 8) will change your life and the way you feel about yourself—and others. Use this tool regularly. Revisit your list often and update it as you need to. Say your top three *out loud* every day and *know* you are *worth* it!

Final Thoughts

This is not the end . . . it's Just the Beginning.

As I mentioned in Chapter 10, the post-detox section, this is just the beginning of your journey. You have just started to dip your toes in the water, and what I want is for you to plunge fully in. This will take time. What is important now is staying on course and being very clear about how you want your life to look and feel moving forward.

If optimal health is something you value, why would you do things that are not in alignment with that? For example, eating doughnuts, not exercising, and indulging in sugary lattes, etc. If you were to enter into a relationship with someone new, and one of your values is kindness, you would not stay with a person who is unkind or mean, would you? That is because your value for kindness is strong and something that you live by.

So what are your health values? Do you have any? Maybe it's time to really get clear, once and for all, what they are. What is your highest vision for yourself when it comes to health and wellness? Where do you see yourself going with all of this new information you have learned? I suggest you get out your journal and write about it now.

Do you want to live a life free of aches, pains, heartburn, indigestion, low energy, moodiness, and other issues? If so, eating and living clean can do that for you. Remember, it's all about prevention, dedication, and education.

I have provided you with a huge education in the pages of this book. Come back and visit it often, use the recipes in your daily life and continue with the exercises I have provided, as I mentioned in the post detox section, Stay the Course: Continuing Practices. This will ensure that you stay on track and that you are aligned with your highest vision and health values.

Remember, it doesn't mean that you can never eat sugar again or drink alcohol, but if optimal health is your highest vision, then why would you want to? Having your list of non-negotiables is key. Make sure you write those down, if you haven't already.

Also, when you live from a place of values and the highest vision you have for yourself, it's not as easy to get caught up in the instant gratification trap. You are clear on what it is that you want for yourself and that overrides any cookie, cake or doughnut in your path. If that is not how you feel right now, you will get there. The longer you engage in positive habits, the more they will become ingrained in your lifestyle.

You have just spent 14 days creating new habits, and it takes time for them to become a part of your wiring in your brain. If you continue on this path with consistency, you will create the new neural pathways that will override the old ones that have kept you stuck in your gooey SAP.

Whatever you decide, I only want the best for you on your journey to an optimally, healthy life. We all have our own way of getting there, and sometimes a little tough love (from yours truly) can help. I get that, sometimes limitations can stand in your way and stop you, and I am here to push you through those limitations, so make sure you visit me often at the Clean in 14 Private Facebook page so I can support you however you need at: on.fb.me/19Daltz

I am honored to be a part of this beautiful journey you have gone on, and excited to be a part of it moving forward.

Remember: You can do anything you put your mind and heart to. If it's important, you will do it, which is why you must be clear on your highest vision for yourself and what your health values truly are.

I am here cheering you on! You are AMAZING!

Resources & Recommendations

Here are some resources that I find very helpful for your continued journey of clean, healthy, plant-based living.

Clean in 14 Bonuses
www.karmachow.com/cleanin14bonuses

A Helpful Website to Research Which Foods to Buy Organic
www.ewg.org/foodnews/

High Quality Supplements, Enzymes and Wellness Support
Pureformulas.com
www.pureformulas.com

Healthy Products
Bob's Red Mill
www.bobsredmill.com
Dried foods, grains, beans, nuts, gluten-free flours

Raw Super Foods
www.essentiallivingfoods.com/
Raw nuts, maca, cacao, nuts

Roasted Dandelion Root Tea
www.traditionalmedicinals.com

Super Foods, Nuts and Seeds
www.navitasnaturals.com
High quality Maca, goji berries, raw cacao

Vegan Protein Powders

Sunwarrior.com

Myvega.com

Amazon.com

Favorite Cookbooks

The Karma Chow Ultimate Cookbook, Melissa Costello.

The Vegan Table, Colleen Patrick Goudreau.

The Hungry Hottie, Cynthia Pasquella.

Veganomicon, Isa Chandra Moskowitz.

Vegan Cooking for Carnivores, Roberto Martin.

Crazy, Sexy Diet, Kris Carr.

Other Books & Films

Sugar Blues, William Dufty.

Eating Animals, Jonathan Safran Foer.

When Food Is Love, Geneen Roth.

Thrive: The Vegan Nutrition Guide to Optimal Performance in Sports and Life, Brendan Brazier.

Thrive Foods: 200 Plant-Based Recipes for Peak Health, Brendan Brazier.

Fat, Sick & Nearly Dead. 2010. Documentary. Written and directed by Joe Cross and Kurt Engfehr. Story by Joe Cross and Robert Mac.

Food, Inc. 2008. Documentary. Directed by Robert Kenner.

Forks Over Knives. 2011. Documentary. Written and directed by Lee Fulkerson.

Hungry For Change, DVD.

Eat to Live: The Amazing Nutrient-Rich Program for Fast and Sustained Weight Loss. Joel Fuhrman.

Vegan for Life: Everything You Need to Know to Be Healthy and Fit on a Plant-Based Diet. Jack Norris and Virginia Messina.

The End of Overeating: Taking Control of the Insatiable American Appetite. David Kessler.

In Defense of Food, Michael Pollan.

Sugar Is Like Heroin. www.ncbi.nlm.nih.gov/pmc/articles/PMC2235907/

Kitchen Gear: Knives, Appliances, Cutting Boards, Etc.

The following are some of my favorite sites that offer high-quality kitchen gear.

Amazon.com

Wayfair.com: Everything you can imagine for your kitchen all on one site!

Sur La Table: High-quality, beautiful, and somewhat pricey selection of every kitchen utensil you can imagine.

Bed, Bath & Beyond: Great for appliances, juicers, cutting boards, glass jars, and storage.

Chef's Catalog.com: An awesome array of chef-quality items.

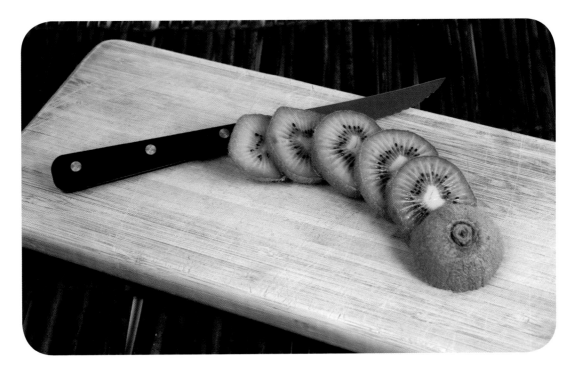

About the Author

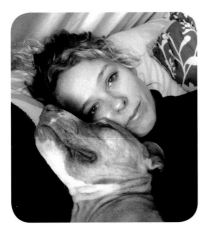

Melissa Costello is a Certified Nutritionist, Wellness Coach, celebrity chef, speaker and author. Her delicious plant-based recipes make living a healthy, preventative life, easy and accessible.

Melissa's passion for plant-based eating brought her to create her company, Karma Chow, as well as the very popular and highly touted *30-Day Vital Life Cleanse,* and the *10-Day Clean Body, Clean Mind Detox,* which was inspiration for this book. She has become the go-to expert in the industry for food-based cleansing.

She is the author of *The Karma Chow Ultimate Cookbook,* and has created recipes, and meal plans for Tony Horton's (P90X) book, *Bring It,* as well as Mandy Ingber's, *New York Times* bestseller, *Yogalosophy.* She is also the host of Beachbody's, Ultimate Reset Cleanse, a 21-day food-based cleanse program.

Melissa has been featured in popular media such as, *TV Guides', Secrets of the Hollywood Body,* Better Life TV, *San Diego Living, Connecticut Style, Orgena Rose Show* and Next Generation TV. She travels extensively across the U.S. speaking at events and educating others on living their best and healthiest life through plant-based eating.

She studied nutrition at NHI in Encinitas, California, and received her certification in wellness coaching through the Spencer Institute. Her certification in Spiritual Psychology from the University of Santa Monica (USM) support her in successfully working deeply with her clients, while helping them to shift sabotaging patterns with food and lifestyle choices that keep them sick, overweight, and unhappy.

Melissa lives in Santa Barbara, California with her sweet pit-bull mix, Pumpkin. She loves to ride horses, hike and spend time at the ocean when she is not creating new, delicious recipes to share with the world.

To learn more about Melissa and her services, visit www.karmachow.com

Alphabetical Recipe Listing

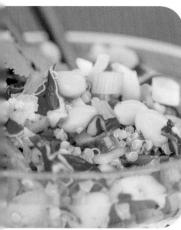

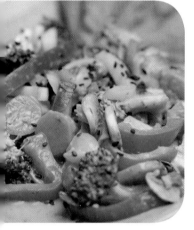

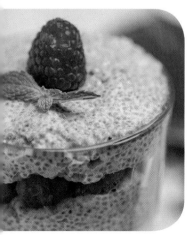

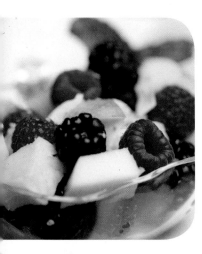

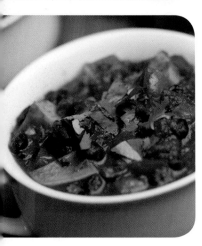

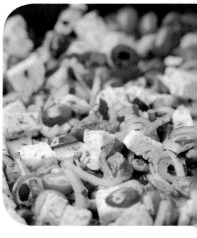

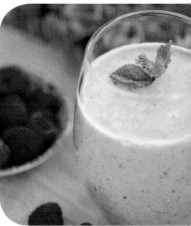

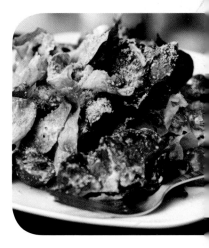

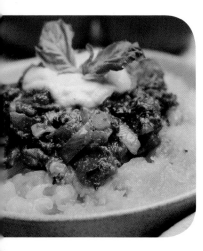

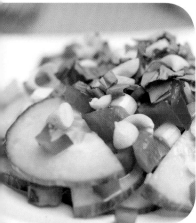

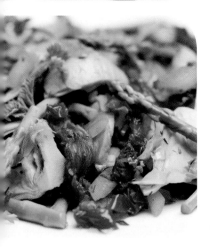

Dressings:

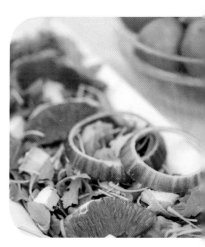

Index